Praise for *Vegan Made Easy*

"*Vegan Made Easy* is more than a book; it's a roadmap to a kinder, healthier, and greener existence. Whether you're a seasoned vegan or a curious explorer, this guide invites you to embrace a lifestyle that celebrates compassion, vitality, and positive change."—**Nancy Arenas**, organizer of Red & Green VegFest, director of Sprouting Compassion; podcast host

"*Vegan Made Easy* is a wonderful, practical how-to guide for anyone interested in going vegan. Especially notable is the underlying message of the book that above all, veganism is a powerful expression of compassion. In providing essential information and easy-to-apply steps for going vegan, Drs. Perussello and Kong show that we are not powerless against the current food system; rather, we can embrace the power of our individual choices to create a kinder and more sustainable world."—**Gene Baur**, co-founder, Farm Sanctuary

"Drs. Perusello and Kong have created a thorough and thoughtful primer for those embarking on a plant-based diet, outlining the philosophy of veganism, the many personal and global health benefits of a plant-based diet, the data behind the impact of the animal agriculture industry on our world, and so much more. In *Vegan Made Easy*, those new to a vegan lifestyle can begin their journey by utilizing the authors' clear and easy-to-understand steps toward a plant-based approach to life. The book is packed with helpful information, including an FAQ section, shopping guides, and many beautiful recipes. Enough to help anyone get started! *Vegan Made Easy* is a great first-step book for anyone interested in learning more about a vegan lifestyle."—**Jennifer Cable**, DMA, singer, voice teacher, qigong and mindfulness practitioner

"*Vegan Made Easy* is a comprehensive guide on how we can invite veganism into our life at a pace that works for us. Importantly, the authors take us on this path in a welcoming and non-judgmental manner. Their book offers solid scientific research as well as reasons why becoming vegan yields such a positive impact on our bodies, the animals, and the planet we all share. They also thoughtfully included a variety of easy and tasty recipes as well as additional resources to help us continue this new, exciting journey."—**Jean L.B. Creamer**, vegan cartoonist

"A source book on all things vegan, this book is a comprehensive, yet succinct treatise on all aspects of veganism and a must read for those venturing into the plant-based lifestyle. A MUST DO for all planetary travelers at this pivotal moment in time."—**Dr. Elisa Beth Haransky-Beck**, Doctor of Optometry specializing in natural eyesight improvement from the inside out; founder, Vegan Spirituality-Southwest PA; author of *Enlivening Consciousness*

"Wow! Just the title, *Vegan Made Easy*, says it all. Not only will you find it easy, but you'll also discover how much more of an impact going vegan makes. Think of how you can make a difference depending on what you purchase. Food, of course, but clothing, furniture, and even cleaning supplies. You'll be amazed at the powerful impact just one person can make. Be one of those who do make a difference."—**Ruth E. Heidrich**, PhD, past president & BOD of The Vegan Society of Hawaii, and author of *A Race For Life*, *Senior Fitness*, *Lifelong Running*, and more

"Dr. Perussello and Dr. Kong's book is perhaps one of the most comprehensive and greatest guides on the how and why of veganism."—**Keegan Kuhn**, filmmaker and co-director of *Cowspiracy* and *What the Health*

"Don't make the mistake of believing that there's anything difficult about going vegan! Just pick up a copy of Camila Perussello and Joanne Kong's *Vegan Made Easy*, and all your questions will be answered, all your doubts resolved, and your motivation to do the right thing for the animals, the planet, and your own body will spike. Let this book be your introduction to a longer and healthier life, lived more sustainably and kindly."—**Glen Merzer**, author of *Food Is Climate*, *Own Your Health*, and *America Goes Vegan!*; co-author of *Chef AJ's Sweet Indulgence*; podcast host

"A wonderful introduction to both the how and why of changing our approach to food—and including the best Q&A on the subject I've seen anywhere—*Vegan Made Easy* is a must-have for the veg-curious. It's also a welcome addition to the library of any vegan who wants to address the concerns of friends and family in a fully educated way."—**Victoria Moran**, author of *Main Street Vegan* and *Age Like a Yogi*

"*Vegan Made Easy* is a timely, engaging, and essential book, deserving a place on everyone's shelf as a reference store of knowledge. The tone is set from the start, with the social justice movement that defines veganism leading the way. Like many new vegans, I once wondered, "Well, what am I going to eat today?" This book has you covered, highlighting research as the key to sustaining your body while protecting and sparing an animal's precious life. You are guided every step of the way, well beyond your diet, to become a true animal hero. Here's to the hope of peace in our time, which only veganism can deliver!"—**Denis Nealis**, organizing volunteer with *Sentient Rights Ireland*

"*Vegan Made Easy* lives up to its title. The authors set the stage for evolving your understanding with the big picture—why it's so important to be vegan. They zoom into many insights for how to be vegan so you can put new directions into practice. Through this book, you'll realize how you can make compassionate, sustainable choices as part of a worldwide community. If you've ever thought about being vegan, this book will be a much-used guide."—**Janice Stanger**, PhD, author of *The Perfect Formula Diet*

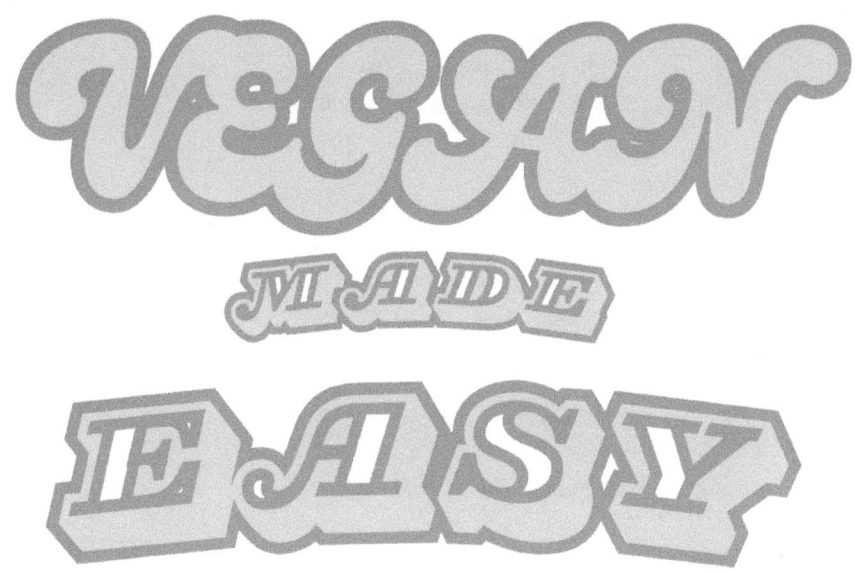

VEGAN MADE EASY

A Practical Guide to Plant-Based Living

Camila Perussello, PhD

and

Joanne Kong, DMA

Foreword by Sailesh Rao, PhD

Lantern Publishing & Media • Woodstock and Brooklyn, NY

2025
Lantern Publishing & Media
PO Box 1350
Woodstock, NY 12498
www.lanternpm.org

Copyright © 2025 Dr. Camila Perussello, PhD, and Dr. Joanne Kong, DMA

All rights reserved. No part of this book may be reproduced, stored in a retrieval system, or transmitted in any form or by any means, electronic, mechanical, photocopying, recording, or otherwise, without the written permission of Lantern Publishing & Media.

Printed in the United States of America

Library of Congress Cataloging in-Publication Data

Names: Perussello, Camila author | Kong, Joanne, 1957- author | Rao, Sailesh author of introduction, etc.
Title: Vegan made easy : a practical guide to plant-based living / Dr. Camila Perussello, PhD and Dr. Joanne Kong, DMA with a foreword by Dr. Sailesh Rao, PhD.
Description: Woodstock, NY ; Brooklyn, NY : Lantern Publishing & Media, 2025. | Includes bibliographical references.
Identifiers: LCCN 2025002892 (print) | LCCN 2025002893 (ebook) | ISBN 9781590567494 paperback | ISBN 9781590567500 epub
Subjects: LCSH: Veganism—Philosophy | Nutrition | Vegan cooking | Diet—Moral and ethical aspects | Animal welfare—Moral and ethical aspects | LCGFT: Cookbooks
Classification: LCC TX392 .P478 2025 (print) | LCC TX392 (ebook) | DDC 641.5/6362—dc23/eng/20250227
LC record available at https://lccn.loc.gov/2025002892
LC ebook record available at https://lccn.loc.gov/2025002893

This book is dedicated to the trillions of animals who
needlessly lose their lives every year.
May readers be inspired to realize the greatest gifts of being
vegan—compassion and gratitude for all life.

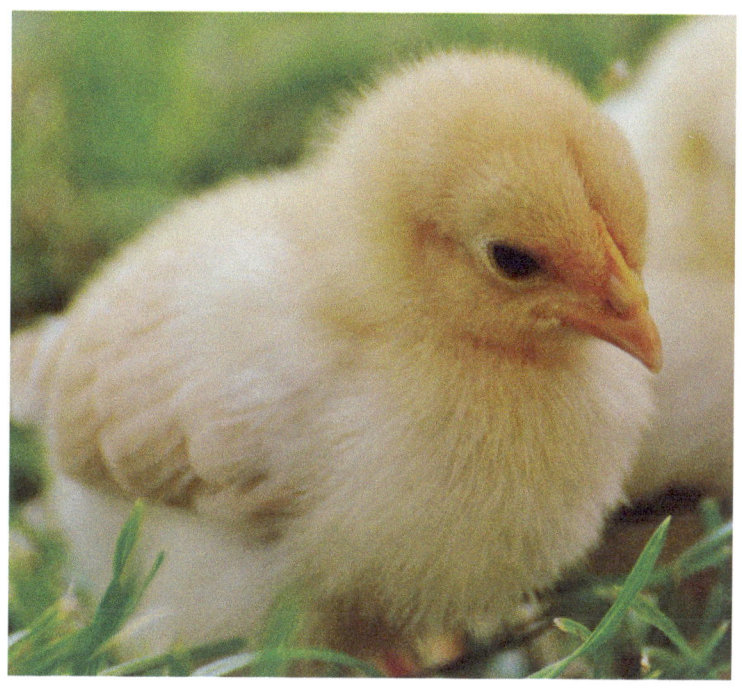

Table of Contents

Foreword by Dr. Sailesh Rao xii
Introduction by Dr. Joanne Kong xvii

Chapter 1—Why Vegan?
    1.1 Social Justice 1
    1.2 Human Health 8
    1.3 Environmental Sustainability 18

Chapter 2—Making the Transition to Plant-based Eating
    2.1 You Already Eat Plant-based Food 29
    2.2 Ways to Make the Transition 30
    2.3 Types of Plant-based Diets, With a Focus on a Whole Food Plant-based Diet 38
    2.4 Making Your Meals Plant-based 42
    2.5 Plant-based Alternatives to Everyday Ingredients 45
    2.6 How to Navigate Social Challenges 52

Chapter 3—Plant-based Food Shopping Guide
    3.1 Eating Plant-based is Cheaper Than Eating Animal Products 59
    3.2 Stocking Your Plant-based Kitchen 62
    3.3 Food Processing: Myths and Truths 69
    3.4 Understanding Food Labels and Ingredients 79
    3.5 Eating Plant-based on a Budget 94

Chapter 4—Veganism Beyond Food
    4.1 Shopping Cruelty-free 100
    4.2 Clothing, Accessories, and Shoes 100
    4.3 Cosmetics, Skincare, and Shampoos 101

4.4 Medicines and Supplements 101
4.5 Cleaning Materials and Detergents 103
4.6 Furnishings 103
4.7 Sports and Entertainment 103

Chapter 5—Frequently Asked Questions
1. Where do I get my protein on a plant-based diet? 105
2. Will I get calcium deficient if I quit dairy? 110
3. Aren't vegans iron deficient? 112
4. Vegans must supplement with B12.
   Doesn't this mean a plant-based diet is unhealthy? 114
5. What plant-based foods are rich in omega-3 and omega-6? 115
6. Is it safe to eat plant-based during pregnancy and lactation? 118
7. Should I take collagen supplements on a plant-based diet? 119
8. I have diabetes. Can I be vegan? 121
9. What are good pre- and post-workout vegan meals? 123
10. My partner will not go vegan. What should I do? 125
11. I eat meat. Why don't vegans understand my diet is a personal choice? ... 126
12. Don't vegans care about plant suffering? 127
13. Why do vegans care more about animals than humans? 129
14. Animals eat animals, so why can't I? 129
15. Do vegans eat eggs from backyard hens? 130
16. I eat free-range meat and eggs. I'm not hurting animals, am I? ... 132
17. I'm vegetarian. I'm not hurting animals, am I? 133
18. Isn't eating local more important than
    eating plant-based to reduce your carbon footprint? 135
19. What will happen to animal farmers if we all go vegan? 137
20. Animal agriculture contributes significantly to the GDP of most nations.
    Is a plant-based food system economically feasible? 138
21. What are some tips for travelling as a vegan? 143
22. It's impossible to be 100% vegan, so why even try? 145

Chapter 6—Recipes

    6.1 Breakfast 152

    6.2 Main Dishes 160

    6.3 Sauces & Sides 184

    6.4 Soups & Breads 188

    6.5 Salads & Sandwiches 197

    6.6 Desserts 206

Chapter 7—Resources

    7.1 Books 216

    7.2 Documentaries 217

    7.3 Websites 218

    7.4 Podcasts 220

    7.5 Apps 221

Final Thoughts by Dr. Camila Perussello 223

References 225

About the Authors

About the Publisher

Foreword

Dr. Sailesh Rao

In our hearts, the world is already vegan, since I haven't met a single person who said that they would deliberately hurt an innocent animal unnecessarily. The only question is how quickly our minds will overcome the gaslighting of the animal agriculture industry and its enablers regarding the age-old nutritional myths that protein is only found in meat, calcium is only found in milk, omega-3 fatty acids are only found in fish, and eating carbs makes you fat, as well as the newest climate myth that cutting down half the trees on the planet had nothing to do with climate change.

Many renowned medical doctors and scientists have been battling nutritional myths for several decades. Many activists have been battling the newest climate myth for over a decade now.

Millions of people are dying every year as a result of these myths. So are trillions of animals and the planet itself. The good news is that the public is now becoming increasingly aware of this industrial gaslighting. A rapidly growing community of around 100 million thriving vegans worldwide is helping to dispel these myths.

In February 2023, the students at Cambridge University voted overwhelmingly for their cafeterias to become 100 percent vegan. In November 2023, the Oxford Union affirmed that "This House Would Go Vegan." In March 2024, the Oxford Literary Festival served whole-food, plant-based vegan meals during the opening and closing gala dinners to standing ovations for the chef, Marlene Watson-Tara.

The younger generation is clearly going vegan full-on. And nothing could be more timely than this comprehensive guide, *Vegan Made Easy*, that Dr. Joanne Kong and Dr. Camila Perussello have written to help people navigate the twists and turns of this transformation from a climate-heating civilization to a climate-healing civilization.

Time is of the essence. Scientists at the Stockholm Resilience Institute estimated that humanity had transgressed three planetary boundaries in 2009, four planetary boundaries in 2015, and six planetary boundaries in 2023. If we fail to pull back within its boundary in a timely manner, any one of these transgressions is sufficient to end life as we know it. Therefore, transgressing six boundaries in our planetary home is like lighting six raging fires in our residential home.

When our home is on fire, we won't be sitting around doing our daily routines, drinking coffee and reading the latest newsfeed on our social media channels. We certainly won't be asking how much gasoline we could pour on the fires or how many lighted cigarette butts we could flip into the fires. Indeed, any sensible person would be joining the bucket brigade and manning the fire hoses to put out the fires.

The vegan movement is that bucket brigade for our beautiful planet. Rewilding the land freed from the erstwhile animal agriculture industry in a climate-healing vegan world is the equivalent of the fire hoses used to put out the planetary fires. Indeed, as the world continues to go vegan, rewilding will free up planetary resources to help put out not one or two, but all six planetary fires.

The least violated planetary boundary transgression is freshwater change. Rewilding the land that is currently used for grazing animals will restore the freshwater cycles of the planet.

The next is land-system change. Going vegan will allow us to return nearly 40 percent of the ice-free land area of the planet back to nature, resolving this planetary-boundary transgression.

The next worst transgression is climate change, which can be resolved when the excess carbon in the atmosphere is absorbed in the three trillion trees and soil that we can restore to the ecosystems of the planet in a vegan world. Indeed, the United Nations estimates that the three trillion standing trees on the planet and the soil that they live on store three times as much carbon as all the fossil fuels we have burned to date or twice as much carbon as that contained in the entire atmosphere. Therefore, with some simple third-grade arithmetic, we can deduce that climate change is completely reversible in a vegan world.

The next is chemical pollution, which would be safely stored away in regenerating forests when we go vegan. Eating animal foods currently delivers concentrated doses of this chemical pollution into our bodies through bioaccumulation. Therefore, going vegan addresses chemical pollution for both the Earth and ourselves.

The next worst transgression is nitrogen and phosphorus loading, mainly through our overuse of synthetic fertilizers for crops. Since over half the crop outputs are fed to farmed animals, going vegan will resolve this transgression as well.

All of these transgressions impact wildlife, and biodiversity loss is the worst of the six planetary-boundary transgressions. By restoring habitats for wild animals and allowing them to live freely in the ocean, we will resolve this transgression as well. If instead we let wild animals die, we die.

Going vegan is therefore a necessary journey, but not a destination. Stopping the consumption of animal products is just the first step in this journey. Dr. Perussello and Dr. Kong are doing a great service to humanity by compiling all the necessary information in an easy-to-read book for anyone embarking on this journey.

This is surely destined to be a well-thumbed book on coffee tables around the world.

Introduction

Dr. Joanne Kong

Plant-based. Vegan. These are words we are seeing more and more, and if you have picked up this book, perhaps you are curious about exactly what it means to go vegan!

In the food context, we are exposed to new information almost daily, whether in the grocery store, in advertisements, online, or by talking with friends or family who may have recently made changes to their diet and lifestyle. Certainly, food choices are some of the most important decisions we make. Each of us has grown up with unique family and cultural traditions, ones we accepted and felt comfortable with. We are all creatures of habit, with a natural tendency to keep things as they have always been. For many, that has included the regular consumption of animals and animal products. So why should one instead consider moving toward plant-based living, and why now?

There are many reasons why the plant-based lifestyle has grown in popularity and appeal, entered mainstream consciousness, and continues to be adopted by growing numbers of people around the globe. For many, the immense health benefits are a primary factor. At a time when we are seeing alarming rises in obesity and the prevalence of so-called Western diseases, aptly described as "diseases of affluence" or, in the United States, the "Standard American Diet (SAD)," the awareness is growing that moving away from using animals as a food source and adopting a diet rich in fruits, vegetables, whole grains, nuts, and seeds are key to enhanced wellness and disease prevention. A new paradigm for good health has emerged, one in which we recognize the power of plant-based eating to provide our bodies with optimal energy and health. Many, including those in the medical profession, also attest to its power to heal and, in numerous instances, reverse disease and long-standing physical ailments. Certainly, there are no guarantees, and every individual has a unique health profile, but plant-sourced nutrition is shown to be strongly advantageous to maintaining good health.

While the terms *plant-based* and *vegan* are often used interchangeably in reference to a plant diet, the latter term points to a deeper significance of not using animals. In its widest sense, it is a philosophy, a way of peaceful living that connects to so many aspects of our lives. As you will learn in this book, going vegan is one of the most powerful things you can do to protect animals from unnecessary suffering, save our environmental resources and wildlife, fight climate change, and help bring about a more sustainable and efficient global food system. It is about restoring the balance between ourselves and the natural world. By turning away from using animals for nourishment, commodities, and entertainment, we expand our capacity for compassion and see that our true nature is grounded in empathy, kindness, and connection to all beings, human and non-human alike. Most importantly, veganism is about justice: it recognizes the intrinsic rights of all living creatures to be free from harm and exploitation.

Like so many others, you may also find that embarking on the plant-based path is an opportunity for self-reflection, increased mindfulness, and even discovering a sense of renewed purpose. Going vegan enlivens our curiosity about the world around us and how we live. It is never about limitations, but rather an opportunity to expand our awareness as we acquire new skills and perceptions, and see food and other animals in a new light. The transition is unique for everyone, and one to be celebrated!

We were motivated to write this book as a guide to exploring veganism and how to go about making the shift in practical, easy ways. You will read about what influences so many to adopt plant-based living, ways to make the transition, and many how-to tips for everything from stocking your vegan kitchen, shopping, understanding food labels, and planning meals, to navigating social challenges and learning about other crucial lifestyle components of vegan living that go beyond diet. An entire chapter is devoted to the most common questions that come up regarding veganism, and a list of numerous resources is included as well. Finally, the book features sample recipes from ten contributors: Nancy Arenas, Chef AJ, Fernando Grando, Jim McGehee, Karoline Mueller, Nancy Poznak, Christoph Wagner, Marlene Watson-Tara, and the authors. These contributors include some of the many influential chefs, culinary instructors, and writers who are inspiring people to embrace the benefits of plant-based eating.

We are fortunate to live at a time when a phenomenal amount of information on veganism is easily accessible, and we hope that this book will be just one of many resources you discover to guide you on your plant-based journey.

Chapter 1

Why Vegan?

1.1 Social Justice

Social justice is the concept that all individuals and groups within a society are deserving of moral consideration and should have their fundamental rights protected. It recognizes and addresses systemic inequalities, discrimination, and injustices based on factors such as race, gender, socioeconomic status, ethnicity, or other characteristics. Social justice aims to create a society where everyone is treated with dignity and respect. Throughout history, we have fought to extend our circle of moral concern. While we are still far from a just society, we have made undeniable progress, especially in the past few centuries.

Even though most people express general opposition to injustice, the extent of their awareness, understanding, and commitment to addressing injustice varies widely. Many among us fail to notice or acknowledge blatant forms of injustice that show up in our everyday lives—and most of those regard our fellow animals, both in quantity and severity.

While violence and discrimination are still commonplace in today's society, no other group of individuals on the planet is treated with more disregard than non-human animals. *Trillions* of living, breathing beings are exploited and killed every year in the food industry alone. Farmers and fishers have the *legal right* to genetically modify, forcefully impregnate, catch, imprison, confine, exploit, buy, sell, mutilate, kill, dismember, profit from, and discard animals like broken machines. Yet, animals are not objects.

Animals are unique individuals who feel, think, and have an obvious interest in avoiding suffering, seeking pleasure, and staying alive—just like us. Animal use represents horrific yet barefaced abuse protected by law.

Discrimination or prejudice based on an individual's species is termed *speciesism*. Speciesism typically favors the interests of one's own species over those of other species. Where have we seen this before? Exactly—everywhere, all the time! The concept of speciesism, often applied to discussions about the ethical consideration of animals, challenges the belief that the interests of humans are inherently more important than the interests of non-human animals. In a speciesist framework, certain species are given preferential treatment, rights, or consideration solely based on their belonging to a particular group. Species discrimination can manifest in various ways, such as using animals for food, clothing, entertainment, or research—but only if they belong to select species. Speciesism prompts reflection on the ethical implications of animal use and how a mature society would treat all sentient beings.

Social justice involves advocating for practices and policies that protect individuals from oppression, discrimination, and abuse, seeking to rectify historical and structural disparities, and fostering a more responsible society. Veganism is an ethical stance opposing the use and oppression of *anyone*, anywhere. Being vegan is recognizing that no one should have the legal entitlement to objectify others.

Education, open dialogue, and empathy can be crucial in promoting individual and collective commitment to addressing injustice and working toward positive social change. When we know better, we can (and should) do better.

Injustice and its Many Forms

Some people may actively engage in social justice efforts, advocating for the rights of marginalized groups and challenging systemic injustices. Others may be less aware of certain expressions of domination and supremacy or hold different opinions about what is unjust. Additionally, there are those who are indifferent to or complacent about injustice due to a belief that they should not care as long as they are unaffected by such issues. Factors such as cultural background, personal experiences, education, societal influences, one's inherent moral compass, and even mental disorders can shape individuals' perspectives on what constitutes injustice and how to address it. However, fostering a greater understanding of various perspectives that enable people to make obvious connections can contribute to building a justice-driven society where unnecessary suffering is avoided and frowned upon.

We have dominated others since the dawn of human civilization, using arbitrary criteria to defend the idea that our lives are somehow more worthy. "Women are born to serve men." "People of color are born to serve white people." "Animals are born to serve humanity." More than ever, we have the knowledge and tools to understand that underneath apparent differences, we all share a common trait: sentience. Sentience is the capacity to feel and be aware of what is happening to and around us. It is the ability to experience pleasure, pain, emotions, and other physical and subjective states. Sentient beings, including human and non-human animals, have awareness and the ability to undergo various mental and emotional states. The concept of sentience is fundamental to discussions about ethical considerations, particularly in animal welfare and rights, as it recognizes the obvious (and extensively proven) fact that animals suffer emotionally and physically.

The animals we use, trap, kill, eat, wear, and experiment on can feel and think; they have a unique personality and interests of their own; they care for their babies, make friends, fear external threats, and hold on dearly to their precious lives. Just for food purposes, an estimated 90 billion land animals and trillions of water animals are subjected to unavoidably cruel practices every single year. *Kind exploitation* is an oxymoron. By mass exploiting and murdering our fellow beings, we miss the opportunity to live by the very same principles we claim to hold and fight for: justice, peace, and empathy.

We cannot possibly build a society that is conscious of the importance of non-harm while we disregard the suffering of the vulnerable—and in such colossal numbers. Our mundane choices, such as what to eat for lunch or what to wear, speak volumes about our core values. Even if unwittingly, every non-vegan reinforces that some lives matter more than others. In fact, each non-vegan contributes to the unnecessary exploitation and killing of hundreds of animals every year—usually by paying other people to hurt and kill on their behalf.

Non-violence is only possible when we are vegan. That is the *beginning* of our journey back to our true selves and unity as opposed to the world of separation, disconnect, and objectification we created for ourselves.

Who Was Your Dinner?

If this question made you uncomfortable, you already understand why veganism is important. In fact, if we all *honestly* reflected on the meaning of these four simple words and acted on them, peace in our society would rise at the drop of a hat. Vegans find it easy not to have chicken for dinner as much as non-vegans find it easy not to have cat for dinner. Like cats and dogs, birds and pigs and cows and fishes and sheep are sentient *individuals*.

Non-vegans usually bring up animal welfare in the conversation, claiming that farmed animals that are well treated and humanely slaughtered do not suffer. Those people are either utterly unfamiliar with animal farming or simply do not care. The thought that there is a justification or a proper way to exploit others is all that is wrong with the world. As animal rights activist Andrea Kladar said on social media, "To examine whether something is humane, first determine if you would want it done to you."

"Happy exploitation" does not exist—especially if you are the victim. Moreover, animal farming involves inherently cruel practices, such as the exploitation of animal bodies and their reproductive cycles. Regardless of the production method, farmed animals are bred into existence to become commodities: females are impregnated against their will to have their offspring, eggs, and breast secretions stolen; babies are separated from their mothers at ridiculously young ages (how does *one day* sound to you?); semen is collected from males through electrical stimulation; female bodies collapse in a fraction of their normal lifespan due to excessive breeding, milking, and egg laying; unprofitable animals are gotten rid of through a shot in the head, gassing, or simply negligence; younger females replace their mothers in the slavery cycle; precious living beings have their worth measured in pounds; and when all of this is over, their life is taken away despite the unmistakable fear in their eyes. Vulnerable creatures cry for our help, yet we use them, wear them, eat them, and flush them down the toilet.

This page may sound like a horror movie. Some may choose to turn the page, throw the book away, or wipe those images from their minds—but what about the animals? They cannot escape our tyranny. Fortunately, you can stop supporting that reality *today* by going vegan. Changing one's lifestyle may seem overwhelming at first, but like any other positive change, *it is worth it*. Remember that if you are reading this book, you have already started. Our purpose is to help readers understand the why and the how behind veganism. Give it a chance, give animals a chance, give *yourself* a chance. There is no greater misery than living in contradiction, and no greater joy than being the best that we can be.

Animal Rights Matter

Among the many justifications used by our species to dismiss the unnecessary suffering inflicted on other beings, some of the most common are tradition, necessity, personal choice, perceived differences in intelligence, and emotional distancing. Let us examine each of them.

- **Tradition**: Animal use and consumption are deeply rooted in cultural traditions. When one justifies abuse in the name of tradition, for consistency, this statement must hold for any other case. Women's oppression, racism, and sexual orientation discrimination are also deeply rooted in cultural traditions. Using tradition as an excuse to dominate others implies that we cannot evolve. Embracing justice, empathy, and the fair treatment of others does not mean cutting ties with our roots; quite the opposite. It means honoring our ancestors and enriching our cultural heritage with ethics and compassion.
- **Necessity**: It is 2025, and there is absolutely nothing we need from other animals to thrive and be happy. Veganism is as old as humanity—the term may well have been coined many decades ago, but millenary religions and peoples have thrived in harmony with other beings. One example is the ancient Indian civilization, particularly during the Vedic period. The concept of *ahimsa*, which translates to non-violence or non-harming, was central to the spiritual and ethical philosophies of various ancient Indian religions, including Hinduism, Buddhism, and Jainism. Even though the ahimsa principle has been overlooked in these religions out of convenience, many practitioners have followed veganism across centuries to minimize harm to other sentient beings.

- **Personal choice**: Every action that intentionally harms others ceases to be a mere personal choice devoid of moral implications. One's favorite color is a personal choice, whether one prefers beach or forest is a personal choice, but depriving others of their dignity and right to live has moral consequences. A small child understands that; why can't we? More on this topic is discussed in Chapter 5, as this is (shockingly) a widespread claim in favor of animal exploitation.
- **Perceived differences in intelligence**: When one claims that humans are entitled to use other animals because they are less intelligent, this implies that one's IQ is a valid criterion to justify abuse. If that were true, how would we view unintelligent people? Would there be justice if some people held more rights than others because they were genetically blessed with a higher intellect? Pigs are proven to be more intelligent than dogs and small children—what would be the implication of this scientific fact if a lower intelligence level justified abuse? If one is not ready to swap their bacon for puppies or toddlers, they should rethink their values.
- **Emotional distancing**: Non-vegans in the Western world are often outraged at cultures that eat dogs. What is the morally relevant justification for eating pigs, chickens, and cows but not dogs? "Dogs are humans' best friends," one would say. We do not know about you, but we do not go around eating anyone who is not our friend. Pigs, cows, chickens, and fishes are social beings who love to play, interact with other species, and have beautiful bonds with humans. Visit an animal sanctuary (even if online) and see the individuals beyond their physical form.

Every single attempt to justify the enslavement, exploitation, or use of animals is easily refuted by a simple exercise of logic. Veganism is all about making obvious connections. Sentience is the only morally reasonable principle on which our treatment of others should be based. Is the victim capable of suffering? That is all we need to ask ourselves.

All sentient beings have the right to be alive, follow their own purpose, and to not be used. The concept of rights is a foundational principle in legal and ethical frameworks, guiding how individuals should be treated within a society. In many legal systems around the world, farmed animals are considered property. They are categorized as commodities or assets owned by individuals, businesses, or entities engaged in agriculture. This legal classification has significant implications for how animals are treated and regarded.

As property, farmed animals are subject to laws governing ownership, transactions, and use. In other words, they are regarded as objects of economic value rather than as beings with inherent rights. In recent years, there has been growing awareness and advocacy for better legal protections for non-human animals. Nonetheless, the property status of farmed animals remains a significant factor in the legal framework surrounding their treatment and rights. Legal changes and discussions are ongoing as society grapples with evolving perspectives on animal ethics. Being vegan is recognizing others' intrinsic rights and, by doing so, accelerating an indeed just society.

Rights, Empathy, and Compassion

Giving animals rights is about mercy or compassion for animals, just as much as giving women rights is about mercy or compassion for women. As individuals, animals (and women) have fundamental rights. Nevertheless, there is an essential relationship between rights, empathy, and compassion.

In the context of human rights, empathy can drive individuals and societies to advocate for the rights of marginalized or oppressed groups. Similarly, in the realm of animal rights, empathy toward non-human animals can inspire efforts to recognize and protect their interests and dignity.

The connection between rights and empathy highlights the moral and ethical dimensions of recognizing and respecting the rights of others. Empathy can motivate social change, influencing individuals and societies to work toward a more just and compassionate world where rights are acknowledged and upheld.

Get to know a farmed animal. Visit a rescue center, volunteer in an animal sanctuary, or (for the brave) watch slaughterhouse videos online. No words are needed when we look an animal in the eye. Make the connection.

We finish this section by highlighting how amazing and fascinating animals are! Everyone who has ever met an animal agrees with that. The animal kingdom is incredibly diverse, and different species display a wide range of complex behaviors. Animals show deep affection for their babies, help each other in times of need, and demonstrate empathy, care, and concern—even toward humans. They have unique personalities, problem-solving abilities, and playfulness. Observing animals in their natural habitats or in human care reveals a rich tapestry of behaviors that showcase their undeniable intelligence, emotional depth, and social connections.

Many people find joy and inspiration in observing animals (we surely do), fostering a sense of appreciation and respect for the diversity of life on Earth. Animals often come into our lives to teach us true love—whoever has a beloved companion animal at home can testify that they really show us what unconditional love is. Very frequently, our relationships with animals are the stepping stones for new relationships with humans after a severe heartbreak. Animal lives are precious!

You do not need to love animals to be vegan, but you need to be vegan to truly love animals.

1.2 Human Health

There is an inside joke among vegans saying that at the mention of veganism, everyone turns into nutritionists, evolutionary anthropologists, and plant advocates. In a health context, everybody seems to know a vegan who allegedly died of a terrible disease because of their diet. In the meantime, cardiovascular diseases (which are closely linked to animal-centered diets) are the top killer in the world. According to the World Health Organization (WHO), heart attacks and strokes are responsible for nearly 20 million human deaths annually (WHO, 2021). In parallel, cancer incidence rates have been increasing sharply over the decades, killing around 10 million people every year (WHO, 2022). The global incidence of early-onset cancer (i.e., occurring in individuals younger than fifty) increased by 79.1 percent between 1990 and 2019 and is projected to increase by another 31 percent by 2030 (Zhao et al., 2023). The rise in cancer incidence can be attributed to several factors, including lifestyle, aging population, environmental factors, improved detection methods, and diet. Colorectal cancer, for instance, is one of the most common cancers worldwide—and one that has been extensively proven to be associated with meat consumption.

A robust (and ever-growing) body of evidence shows that balanced plant-based diets offer numerous health benefits. Rich in fruits, vegetables, whole grains, legumes, nuts, and seeds, this dietary approach is associated with lower risks of chronic conditions such as heart disease, hypertension, and type 2 diabetes. The abundance of fiber, vitamins, minerals, and antioxidants in plant foods supports digestive health, enhances immune function, reduces body inflammation, and provides a wide range of nutrients essential for overall well-being. Research also links plant-based diets to weight management, improved cholesterol levels, better hormonal balance, and a reduced risk of cancer overall.

Despite irrefutable evidence, misconceptions about the health benefits of vegan diets are widespread due to a combination of factors. First, there is a general lack of understanding about what constitutes a plant-based diet and how diverse and rich it can be. Second, poor nutritional knowledge among the population contributes to misconceptions, as not everyone possesses a deep understanding of how to eat healthily, let alone on a vegan diet. Additionally, decades-long propaganda by the animal agriculture industry and widespread use of their products (starting with school cafeterias) ingrained in our minds the idea that animal products are healthy and necessary. Media influence, often oversimplifying or sensationalizing nutrition information, further contributes to this confusion. Another critical component of the misinformation on plant-based eating is the stigmatization of veganism as a whole. When confronted with their moral inconsistencies, non-vegans commonly choose to attack veganism instead of acknowledging that their choices harm animals. A frequent way to deflect the conversation and avoid inner reflection is by questioning different elements of veganism, including plant-based eating—even if this means going against undeniable facts and scientific evidence.

Ironically, half-truths and outright lies are increasing in the era of information due to the rapid dissemination of ideas facilitated by digital platforms and social media. Influencers and cheap tabloids often spread misinformation about veganism and plant-based eating to capitalize on sensationalism and controversy. By presenting misleading, one-sided, or exaggerated narratives about veganism, these publications tap into existing biases or skepticism, fostering polarized and factually inaccurate discourses. The prioritization of clickable headlines over factual accuracy, coupled with controversy and the reinforcement of negative stereotypes, serves the tabloids' goal of maximizing profits through increased circulation and advertising revenue. A lack of literacy skills and critical thinking, along with intentional disinformation campaigns, further exacerbates the problem. The focus on attention-grabbing stories leads to the propagation of inaccurate information that hinders serious discussions about the ethical, environmental, and health aspects of veganism. The result? *Everyone* loses.

Sadly, medical doctors can also fall victim to incorrect information on plant-based diets. While most physicians prioritize evidence-based medical advice, occasional instances of misinformation about the health impact of veganism from individual doctors may arise due to a variety of factors. These can include the general lack of nutrition education during medical training, personal biases, a lack of up-to-date information on plant-based diets, sensationalized media coverage, and the influence of industry interests. Ideally, healthcare professionals should be knowledgeable about nutrition and the mounting body of scientific evidence supporting the health benefits of plant-based diets.

The following pages summarize the positive health outcomes of the whole-food plant-based (WFPB) diet. The information presented here is based on peer-reviewed studies published in reputable scientific journals. We fully encourage readers to refer to the actual studies in the references section, and to also keep in mind that these represent a tiny fraction of the current research demonstrating the benefits of plant-based diets.

Heart Health

- The WFPB diet is significantly lower in saturated fats and trans fats, higher in poly-unsaturated fats, and cholesterol-free. This helps reduce blood LDL cholesterol levels, providing cardiovascular protective effects (Wang et al., 2023).

- As plant foods are frequently lower in sodium and higher in potassium, healthy plant-based diets can reduce blood pressure and the risk of cardiovascular diseases (Wang et al., 2023; Zarantonello & Brunori, 2023).

Digestive Health and Weight Management

- Whole plant foods are generally lower in calories and higher in fiber, aiding in weight management through the promotion of satiety and faster stool transit (Wang et al., 2023).
- By helping prevent constipation and straining during defecation, a WFPB diet reduces the risk of hemorrhoids, leaky gut syndrome, and other bowel disorders, such as diverticulitis (Nath & Singh, 2017).
- Micronutrients in the WFPB diet lead to lower body inflammation and modulation of the gut microbiota, meaning higher counts of beneficial bacteria and lower counts of pathogenic microorganisms. Extensive research shows that a balanced gut microbiota helps with weight management and overall health (Sakkas et al., 2020). Studies have also been exploring the role of gut microbiota in the development and progression of cancer, including digestive and prostate cancer (Matsushita et al., 2023).

Diabetes Prevention and Control

- Increased fiber ingestion and the nutrient content of plant-origin foods may improve insulin sensitivity and blood sugar control in individuals with diabetes, helping manage and sometimes curing type 2 diabetes (Wang et al., 2023).
- A WFPB diet eliminates the risk factors for type 1 and type 2 diabetes associated with compounds exclusive to animal products. For instance, animal proteins, growth factors, and sexual hormones (e.g., estrogen and progestins in milk) can induce the secretion of insulin and insulin-like growth factor 1 (IGF-1) (Wang et al., 2023; Thomas et al., 2023).

Inflammation Reduction

- Vitamins, minerals, fibers, mono- and poly-unsaturated fats, phytochemicals, and other nutrients abundant in a WFPB diet are linked to lower levels of

inflammation in the body, reducing the risk and severity of chronic inflammatory conditions, from acne and psoriasis to inflammatory bowel disease (IBD) and beyond (Aghasi et al., 2019; Fusano, 2023).
- A WFPB diet is rich in compounds like polyphenols, phytoestrogen, and polyunsaturated fatty acids, which are known to reduce oxidative stress and inflammation in the human body. As chronic inflammation can disrupt hormonal systems, the anti-inflammatory nature of plant foods may positively impact varied hormone-related conditions, such as acne, dermatitis, polycystic ovary syndrome (POS), and others (Chavez et al., 2023; Fusano, 2023).
- Chronic inflammation is associated with an increased risk of obesity, cancer, and a wide range of other health conditions. Although further research is needed, inflammation biomarkers are typically lower in individuals following plant-focused diets, such as C-reactive protein (CRP) and proinflammatory cytokines (Menzel et al., 2020; Thomas et al., 2023).

Cancer-risk Reduction
- A plant-based diet is associated with a lower risk of cancer, especially (but not limited to) digestive cancer, such as colon, rectal, esophageal, pancreatic, stomach, and liver (Huang et al., 2021; DeClercq et al., 2022; Guéraud et al., 2024). Several substances are involved in diet-related cancer development, including synthetic food additives, heavy metals, veterinary drug residues, pesticide residues, dioxins, cancer-promoting compounds naturally found in animal products (e.g., heterocyclic amines), natural and synthetic animal hormones (e.g., estrogen, estradiol, progesterone, testosterone), saturated fats, trans fats, and others. Such compounds are *massively* minimized in a WFPB diet.
- Compounds commonly found in meat (both unprocessed and processed) in significant concentrations, such as HCAs, polycyclic aromatic hydrocarbons (PAHs), and N-Nitroso compounds (NOCs), are associated with an elevated risk of cancer, especially of digestive organs. Some studies suggest that exposure to hormones, particularly those found in dairy products, may increase the risk of breast cancer and prostate cancer (Wang et al., 2023; Melnik et al., 2023). Other components found in dairy milk, such as animal proteins,

- exosomal microRNAs, aflatoxin M1, bisphenol A, residues of pesticides and veterinary drugs, and micro- and nanoplastic, also pose potential cancer risks (Melnik et al., 2023).
- Despite the health-promoting effects of fatty acids and other nutrients found in fish, fish consumption has been associated with a higher risk of skin cancer (both malignant melanoma and melanoma *in situ*), possibly due to environmental contaminants such as mercury and polychlorinated biphenyls (PCBs) (Li et al., 2022).
- Although more research is warranted for individual animal products and cancer types, current evidence on the relationship between meat intake and cancer is abundant and strong (WHO & IARC, 2015; Huang et al., 2021; Guéraud et al., 2024). Based on a careful assessment of *hundreds* of peer-reviewed studies, the WHO and the International Agency for Research on Cancer (IARC) classified processed meat (e.g., bacon and ham) as a Group 1 carcinogen (the top class) and red meat (e.g., steak) as a Group 2A carcinogen (WHO & IARC, 2015). Red meat, especially processed, is linked to increased cancer risk, including colon, breast, endometrium, and other types of cancer (Dunneram et al., 2019; Huang et al., 2021; DeClercq et al., 2022; Guéraud et al., 2024). Besides WHO and IARC, several governments and health organizations worldwide are promoting a reduction in meat consumption as part of their dietary guidelines to combat cancer, including the American Cancer Society, the US Dietary Guidelines, and the UK National Health Service.
- It is worth noting that research on particular types of cancer as a result of the intake of specific foods or dietary patterns is not entirely conclusive, as the studies often differ in design, population characteristics, and methodologies, leading to conflicting findings. For example, the definition of *plant-based diet* is not standardized among studies. Many of them do not differentiate between vegetarian and vegan diets and even include animal flesh in what they consider a plant-based diet. In addition, some studies include individuals who have been following plant-based diets for a short period after being omnivores for a long time, which strongly clouds the conclusions. Also, studies often fail to consider the differences between healthy and unhealthy plant-based diets. It is not fair to

compare a WFPB diet to a junk food vegan diet replicating the Western way of eating. Also, other lifestyle factors beyond diet play a role in cancer risk.
- As discussed in a previous item, chronic inflammation is considered a "hallmark of cancer." While scientists continue unravelling the intricate connections between inflammation and cancer development, modern research shows reduced inflammation markers among people reducing or eliminating the consumption of animal products (Wang et al., 2023). Monitoring inflammation markers is part of ongoing research to identify the best diets for cancer prevention and treatment.

Kidney Disease Prevention and Mitigation

- Studies show that plant-based diets can protect against the onset and evolution of chronic kidney disease. The beneficial effects are ascribed to several factors that protect the kidneys, such as blood pressure regulation, reduced protein intake, and higher intake of antioxidant compounds that lower body inflammation. Notably, plant-based diets offer more advantages than low-protein diets that include animal products (Zarantonello & Brunori, 2023).

Hormonal Balance and Fertility

- A WFPB diet may contribute to better hormonal balance for several reasons. Firstly, plant-based diets are typically rich in fiber and antioxidant compounds, which can play a role in modulating hormonal levels. Fiber helps regulate blood sugar levels, which in turn influences insulin secretion and sensitivity, contributing to better metabolic health. Additionally, plant-based diets are associated with lower levels of saturated fats, trans fats, naturally occurring animal hormones, and synthetic hormones administered to farmed animals. The presence of phytoestrogens in some plant foods also has mild estrogenic effects that may contribute to hormonal balance (Wang et al., 2023).
- Globally, infertility affects an estimated 15 percent of reproductive-age couples trying to conceive. Diets rich in cholesterol, saturated fats, and animal hormones negatively impact the fertility of both men and women due to various factors, including higher visceral fat levels and dysregulation of sex hormones.

A well-planned plant-based diet can contribute to improved fertility, although the impact can vary among individuals and underlying causes of fertility issues. Among the benefits of plant-based diets, weight management, nutrient density, anti-inflammatory effects, improved blood flow, and hormonal balance may exert a positive impact on the health of reproductive organs, semen quality, and overall fertility (Skoracka et al., 2020; Łakoma et al., 2023).

Women's Health and Men's Health

- Plant-based diets may offer potential benefits for women with polycystic ovary syndrome (PCOS) and premenstrual syndrome (PMS), though individual responses can vary. A WFPB diet may help regulate hormonal imbalances associated with PCOS, thanks to the balanced nutrient profile and anti-inflammatory properties of plant foods. For those experiencing PMS, the nutrients and antioxidant compounds of plant-based foods may help alleviate bloating and mood swings (Barnard, 2020).
- While research on this topic is limited, some evidence suggests that plant-based diets may alleviate menopausal symptoms for some women. Plant-based diets rich in fruits, vegetables, whole grains, and legumes may offer benefits due to their high fiber content, anti-inflammatory properties, and the presence of phytoestrogens, which can lessen symptoms associated with declining estrogen levels during menopause. These components may help reduce hot flashes and mood disturbances, as well as mitigate changes in body composition (Barnard, 2020).
- Growing research suggests that the risk of prostate cancer may be lower in men who limit or eliminate the intake of animal foods. This is attributed to reduced exposure to cancer-promoting substances in animal products, as well as a healthier gut microbiota, which positively affects inflammation and testosterone metabolism (Matsushita et al., 2023).

Brain Health

- Robust evidence associates healthy plant-based diets with a lower risk of vascular dementia, Alzheimer's disease, and other types of cognitive decline.

A healthier gut microbiota and nutrients such as phytochemicals and polyunsaturated fatty acids help protect the brain from oxidative stress and inflammation in people following a WFPB diet, contributing to cognitive health (Ding et al., 2022).

Stronger Immune System and Longevity

- Plant-based diets are associated with a longer lifespan. The longevity effects are attributed to a combination of factors, such as lower exposure to environmental toxins built up in animal products; a reduced intake of specific amino acids, saturated fats, and cholesterol; a higher intake of antioxidants; and a healthier gut microbiota (Herpich et al., 2022; Wang et al., 2023; Thomas et al., 2023). Additional factors commonly present among people who eat more mindfully further contribute to their mental and physical health, such as physical activity, meditation, drug abstinence, contact with nature, ethical principles, and purposeful work.

We understand that reading scientific articles may not be realistic (or fun) for everybody—although they are the most reliable source of information we have at hand. For additional clarification regarding health and plant-based diets, we recommend the book *Eating Plant-Based: Scientific Answers to Your Nutrition Questions* (Kassam & Kassam, 2022). This an easy-to-read Q&A book written by two medical doctors with decades of clinical experience.

Despite the many benefits of plant-based eating, please bear in mind that turning vegan does not make you immune to all diseases. While a well-balanced vegan diet can contribute to overall health and well-being, genetics, lifestyle choices, and environmental exposure also play significant roles in determining an individual's health and susceptibility to mental and physical diseases. For example, even though vegans are significantly less susceptible to severe COVID-19 symptoms (Kim et al., 2021), communicable diseases (those caused by pathogenic viruses and bacteria) can affect anyone. Moreover, it is naïve to assume that a plant-based diet will automatically erase decades of poor eating habits and other factors contributing to health conditions. If you have smoked, used drugs, or suffered from bulimia for years, please do not blame your newly adopted plant-based diet for reported health conditions. It sounds silly, but stories like those pop up all the time—and make headlines.

Furthermore, a WFPB diet aligns with sustainable eating, making it beneficial for both personal and environmental health. Multiple studies demonstrate that plant-based eating is the *most effective* way of reducing the global disease burden while combating food insecurity and curbing the environmental crisis. More details are discussed in the next section.

Many people perceive the climate and ecological crises as not directly concerning or affecting them for a combination of reasons, like lack of awareness, delayed impact, psychological distance, short-term interests, and even cognitive dissonance. However, it is not hard to understand that it is impossible to be healthy in an unhealthy environment. A surrounding environment marked by factors such as pollution, extreme weather events, water shortages, limited access to nutritious food, and high stress levels can contribute to physical and mental health challenges. For instance, animal farms increase air pollution through the release of substances like ammonia, particulate matter from animal waste, and animal dander. These airborne pollutants can exacerbate respiratory problems in humans working on or living near animal farms, contributing to conditions like asthma and bronchitis. Recent research demonstrated that a shift away from animal-sourced foods could save USD 7.3 trillion worth of diseases and ecosystem degradation while curbing greenhouse gas (GHG) emissions (Lucas et al., 2023).

Education to promote a deeper understanding of the intrinsic link between human health and the planet's health is essential in fostering a sense of shared responsibility and urgency in addressing the ecological crisis. It is also important to understand that humans are not the only or most relevant species on Earth. Humans have lived on the planet for a ridiculous 0.0066 percent of Earth's history. Valuing and preserving diverse life forms contributes to everyone's well-being and acknowledges the intrinsic worth of each life, fostering a deeper appreciation for the complexity and beauty of the natural world—of which we are all a part.

1.3 Environmental Sustainability

As we look at our world today, those of us possessing only a passing awareness of current events will acknowledge that we are facing unprecedented dangers connected to climate change and environmental damage to our planet. The evidence is there every day, in record-breaking temperatures, devastating hurricanes, flooding and storms, worsening drought conditions, deadly wildfires, rising sea levels and ocean acidification, and water shortages spreading around the globe, all of which threaten the Earth's ecosystems and the survivability of its inhabitants. Humankind has reached its point of greatest damage to the planet, and honest assessments and bold actions are crucial if we are to have a sustainable future.

The challenges we currently face can be traced to the evolution of our relationships with nature and other animals over the long history of human culture. Our early ancestors *coexisted* with the environment, highly observant of animals' unique abilities and fascinated by the powers they seemed to hold. But as nomadic lifestyles gave way to agriculture and the ownership of land and animals, perceptions shifted. Animals became objectified as commodities, and with the ultimate rise of urbanization and consumerism in the modern era, we grew further and further from seeing them as sentient, feeling individuals. They became units of production within industries prioritizing efficiency, profit, and unrestrained economic growth. We have also lost our deep connections and kinship with the environment, bringing widespread depletion and destruction to our precious natural resources. This damage has increased as a slow-moving crisis, distant from our everyday awareness and concerns.

> It is not the dramatic, sudden kind of killing and destruction as that of an all-out nuclear war, but it is killing and destroying: slowly, silently, steadily. . . . We turn prairies into deserts to raise more cattle, sheep, and goats. We turn rainforests into croplands to feed more factory-farmed animals to sate ever-increasing demand for meat and dairy products worldwide. . . . We are changing the world, and not for the better. (Mason, 2021)

Significantly, humanity's use of animals as a food source is central to the escalating threats to our sustainability. Discussions of climate and environmental crises typically center around decarbonizing our energy and transportation systems and moving faster toward renewable energy sources. While these are important parts of the solution, the widespread devastation of animal agriculture remains mostly overlooked, even at the highest levels of governance. It *is* the most destructive industry on the planet today, and one that is massively inefficient. The process of raising and killing animals for food connects to broadscale global concerns, everything from land and fossil fuel use, GHG emissions, pollution, and water and soil depletion, to massive deforestation, ocean destruction, and species and habitat loss. Such negative impacts will only continue to grow, with the world's population expected to reach 10 billion by 2050, and projections that on our current path, the level of meat consumption in 2050 will easily double that of 2008 (The World Counts, 2023). Concerns are on the rise regarding the growing threats of antibiotic resistance and the possibility of more-deadly pandemics in the future, with the global health disaster of COVID-19 serving as a dire warning that we have grown out of balance with the natural world. How ironic it is that our ways of producing food, meant to nourish and sustain us, are now threatening our very existence.

Our survivability will ultimately depend upon accepting the fact that we have arrived at a point of global crisis, and then taking actions that will make a difference. This can be challenging, for human nature is such that we find stability and security in accepting the status quo, continuing the traditions of society we grew up with. There is a natural tendency to resist change, and we can feel apathetic or powerless to tackle large-scale problems that seem disconnected from the concerns of our everyday lives. However, in the matter of food and lifestyle choices, each and every one of us *can* contribute to impactful change. Every single time we eat a plant-based meal or choose not to take part in the exploitation of animals is a powerful statement invested in the belief that a kinder and more sustainable world is possible. The beauty of it is that we do not need to wait for world leaders to create positive change; we can take action as individuals *right now*, as summed up by the saying, "Your plate is the world's fate." A global shift to plant-based eating is essential to the future of our planet (World Economic Forum, 2021).

Let's now examine the negative impacts of the animal agriculture industry.

Land and Fossil Fuel Use

It is critical to examine how the world's food habits intersect with land use. Certainly, humans rely on the productivity of land to feed and nourish a rapidly growing global population. However, the prevailing acceptance of using animals for food relies on using a disproportionate amount of land relative to the resulting nutritive value. While meat and dairy industries use 83 percent of farmland, they yield only 18 percent of the world's calories (Poore & Nemecek, 2018).

By making a decisive global shift toward consuming plant foods instead of growing massive amounts of feed for animals, we would not have to grow as many crops and could free up around 40 percent of the ice-free land area of the planet, as illustrated in Figure 1.

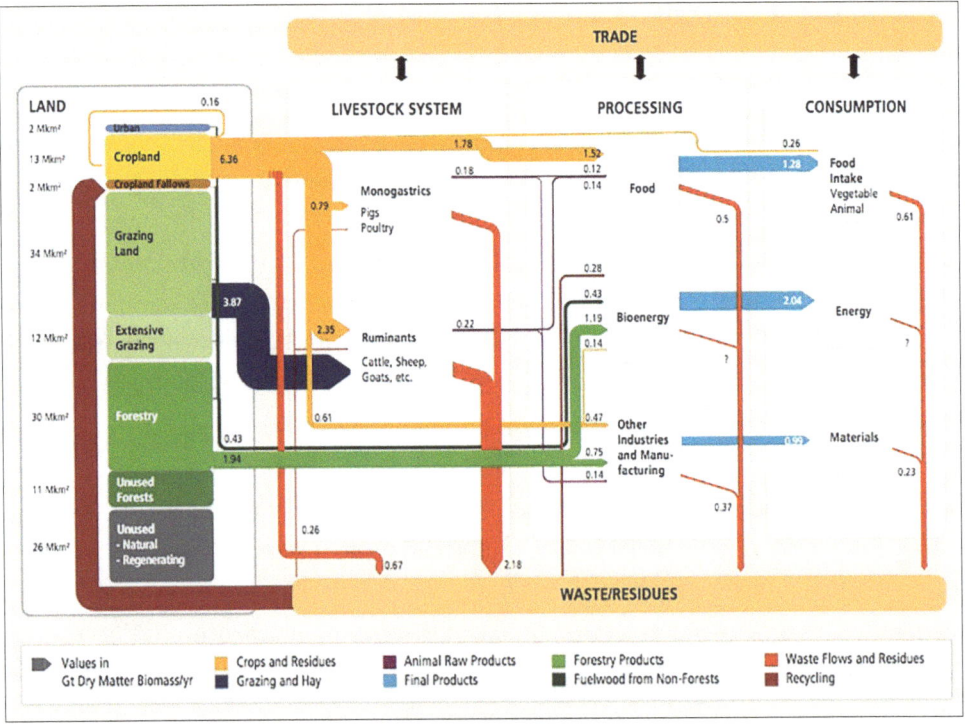

Figure 1. *Land use and observed climate change. Source: IPCC (2019).*

This is critical in addressing the global issue of close to a billion people suffering from chronic hunger. Half of the crops grown worldwide go to livestock instead of to the people who need them the most. In the United States, an astounding 41 percent of land is dedicated to livestock, as seen in Figure 2 (Leatherby & Merrill, 2018).

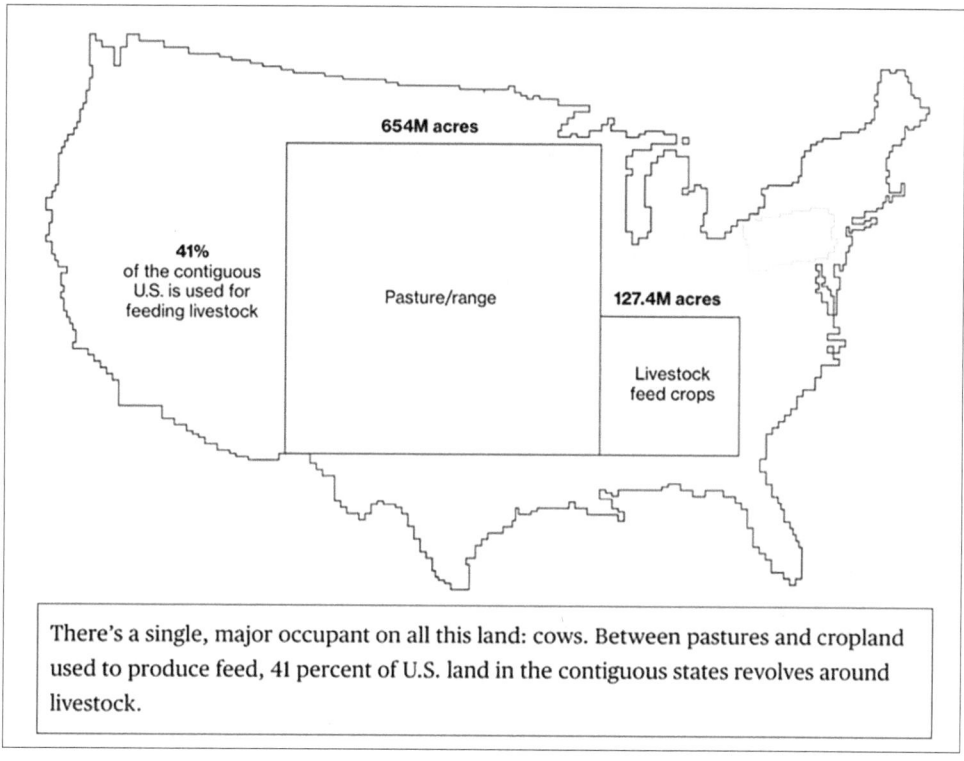

Figure 2. *Use of land for livestock production in the United States. Source: Leatherby & Merrill (2018).*

It is also important to note the inherent inefficiency of using animals as a food source. Farmed animals eat huge amounts of plant food over their short lifespans. For humans consuming those animals, at least 70 percent of the plant's energy is *lost* through the animal's metabolic processes and waste, making us *secondary* consumers of those plants. Instead, it is far more efficient to gain nutrition from the source and eat plants directly. In fact, studies show that we could meet the nutritional needs of 10 billion people if the world went plant-based (Springmann et al., 2018a; Berners-Lee et al., 2018).

The inefficiency of raising animals for food also ties significantly to fossil fuel use (Figure 3). Prevailing discussions, even at the highest levels of global policy, tend to focus on reductions of fossil fuels in transportation and energy systems, ignoring the significantly lower energy footprint of eating plants directly. The typical consumer is unaware of the immense resources that go into animal products, from growing animal feed, raising the animals, feeding them, and running slaughterhouse facilities, to processing, packing, refrigeration, and transportation.

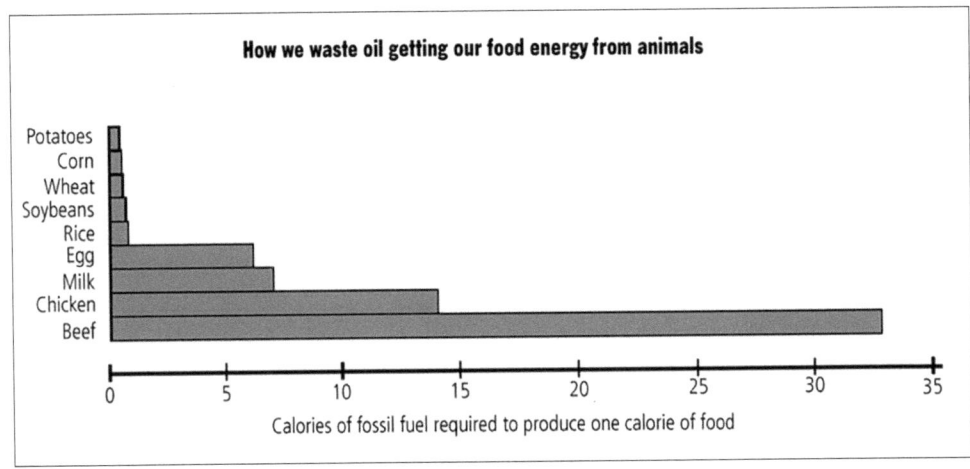

Figure 3. *Food calories produced per calorie input from fossil fuel. Source: Pimentel (1979).*

Climate Change

Our meat-centric culture is a primary driver of climate change. Evidence suggests that animal agriculture easily accounts for over half of global GHG emissions, including carbon dioxide, nitrous oxide, and methane. Estimates vary depending on the considered time frame and important factors disregarded in past studies (FAO, 2006; Goodland & Anhang, 2009; Reisinger & Clark, 2018; Rao, 2021; Eisen

& Brown, 2022). Despite divergences, animal agriculture is established as a leading GHG source and the top driver of methane and nitrous oxide emissions. Often overlooked, methane's global warming potential (GWP) in a five-year period is one hundred times more potent than that of carbon dioxide. It is startling to realize that the climate-changing emissions of the animal agriculture industry surpass those of *all* modes of transportation combined worldwide (FAO, 2006). Figure 4 shows the differences in emissions between animal and plant foods.

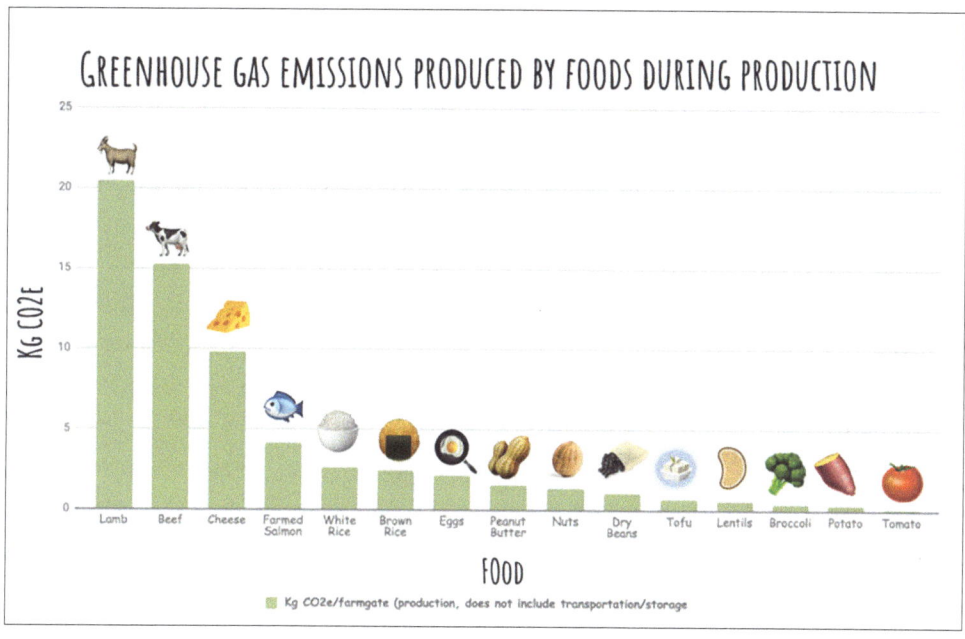

Figure 4. *Greenhouse gas emissions produced by foods. Source: Baker (2018).*

Depletion of Water Resources

The rise in dangerous drought conditions and desertification due to global warming is exacerbated by the vast water footprint of our food systems, in particular, animal agriculture. For an industry that kills billions and billions of land animals every year, the water demands are staggering, with at least a third of agricultural water usage taken up by meat and dairy.

Producing a pound of beef takes an astounding 2,000 gallons of water (Water Footprint Calculator, 2023), at least twenty times the amount needed to grow the equivalent amount of plant foods. Water for animals to drink as well as for maintenance and cleaning of factory farms and slaughterhouses makes up only a small percentage of the total water used to raise animals. Approximately 98 percent is directed to growing animal feed crops (Mekonnen & Hoekstra, 2010). The inefficient use of our precious land, energy, and water resources by raising animals for food clearly must be addressed; as noted earlier, livestock accounts for only 18 percent of the world's calories.

Pollution, Contamination, and Soil Degradation

The animal agriculture industry is a direct contributor to contamination, from enormous amounts of manure, antibiotics, hormones, and chemical fertilizers, to toxic gases, herbicides, and pesticides released into the environment. These substances are a continuing threat to wildlife, plant life, and ecosystems. In the United States, over 200 million pounds of pesticides per year are sprayed on crops grown for livestock (WAP). Clearly, environmental regulations should be stricter, especially those pertaining to factory farms.

Healthy soils, critical to the global food system, are increasingly depleted and degraded due to overgrazing, intensive agricultural production, and monocrop cultures, exacerbated by drought and urban expansion. Roughly 85 percent of soil erosion in the United States is due to grazing, and the United Nations warns that up to 40 percent of the Earth's land is now seriously degraded (Woldeab, 2019; UNCCD, 2022).

Deforestation

Furthermore, unprecedented deforestation is due to animal agriculture, with beef production responsible for 41 percent of forest destruction as lands are acquired for grazing and growing feed crops (Ritchie, 2021b). A recent investigation by the Bureau of Investigative Journalism (TBIJ), the *Guardian*, Repórter Brasil, and Forbidden Stories has shown that the massive loss of forests in the Amazon due to cattle farming has amounted to more than 800 million trees being destroyed in just the past six years (Wasley et al., 2023). Forests are essential to curbing the climate crisis as they absorb a significant portion of the GHGs released from fossil fuel burning and other activities. Not only is stored carbon released as rainforest trees are cut down, worsening climate change, but precious wildlife habitats are also lost. We must bring massive deforestation to an end and focus on restoring and protecting natural ecosystems and habitats. Studies show that plant-based diets can halve forest destruction and prevent up to 78 percent of carbon emissions (Weindl et al., 2017).

Ocean Destruction

Human activity has led to severe impacts on marine life and ecosystems, exacerbated by ocean acidification and rising sea temperatures. We have brought massive destruction to ocean life through overfishing, and about 40 percent of the animals caught are bycatch—sea life unintentionally caught, including turtles, dolphins, whales, sharks, and others. Almost a third of fish populations have now collapsed (Greenpeace, undated). Huge ocean trawlers and discarded fishing nets also cause significant environmental damage, especially to fragile coral reefs and other marine habitats.

Farmed fish is no better. Over half of seafood now comes from aquaculture, comprising fish pens on both land and water:

> Fish farming tends to be grossly inefficient, with more fishes used as feed than produced. It is also egregiously inhumane. The fishes are kept in crowded pens that are polluted with feces and decomposing feed. Diseases can quickly spread through the pens, so antibiotics and other chemicals are heavily used. The captive fishes are often heavily infested with parasitic sea lice, and procedures to get rid of them can be lethal to the fishes. Ocean-based fish farms pollute the surrounding water, and lice and disease can be transmitted through the caging to wild fishes. As with wild-caught fishes, slaughter methods for farmed fishes are brutal and can prolong their suffering. (Finelli, 2021)

Ocean destruction and animal rights violations among aquatic animals are frequently overlooked, even in the vegan movement. More information can be found in *Food for Thought: Planetary Healing Begins on Our Plate* (Perussello, 2022), which has a chapter dedicated entirely to fishes. Organizations such as Fish Feel (www.fishfeel.org) and Sentient Media (www.sentientmedia.org) are helping to dispel the myths that fishes are unfeeling and do not feel pain. Awareness is also growing that fish can no longer be considered a "healthy" food, due to microplastics and ocean contaminants (especially mercury) that are highly concentrated in fish flesh, and dangerously high levels of omega-6 fatty acids compared to omega-3s. The best thing that consumers can do is leave fishes off their plates!

Species and Habitat Loss

Animal agriculture, both of land animals and fish, is a leading cause of species and habitat loss, contributing to the greatest negative environmental impacts on the global food system (Harwatt et al., 2022). More than 107 billion humans have lived on Earth, yet *every* single year, we kill at least 80 billion land animals and trillions of sea animals for food (Francione, 2022). Scientists state we are in the sixth mass extinction, aptly named the Anthropocene, due to human activity. This stunning loss of biodiversity, which at current rates would take 3–5 million years to recover (McCarthy & Sánchez, 2018), threatens the survivability, adaptability, and resiliency of all living beings. It is astounding to realize that even though humans account for only 0.01 percent of the Earth's biomass, we are responsible for the loss of 83 percent of wild mammals (Bar-On et al., 2018). Biodiversity loss is not an issue without consequence, for the diversity of ecosystems is vital to species adaptability, resilience, and survival against environmental changes. All life systems on Earth exist in a complex, interconnected web of existence.

Environmental Racism

The damaging impacts of animal agriculture extend to those living in communities near slaughterhouse facilities. These populations, often low-income people of color, suffer disproportionate amounts of serious health issues, including asthma, bronchitis and other respiratory issues, headaches, burning eyes, and elevated cancer rates. Recent research demonstrates that plant-based diets can reduce air pollution, preventing around 240,000 deaths per year globally (Springmann et al., 2023). Excess manure from huge animal waste pits is often sprayed out over surrounding neighborhoods, as recounted here in an interview with Naeema Muhammed, co-director of the North Carolina Environmental Justice Network:

I see the spraying going on. I see the hog houses and the open-air lagoons that's just sitting out there. [. . .] There are pipes running underneath the ground. And the waste is piped out into the open-air lagoon. And there are all kinds of chemicals. And this urine and fecal matter produces methane, ammonia gases, and so you can smell it. And what people say, it smells like rotten eggs, sometimes rotten collard greens or—it's just a terrible smell. And they have been forced off of their wells, because they were seeing remnants of the waste in their well waters by the coloring and the odors coming out of their well water. (Muhammed, 2017)

It is not only the hazardous environment surrounding these facilities; an often overlooked aspect of the industry is the systemic victimization endured by workers. Many are grossly underpaid and undocumented immigrants, suffering a rate of severe injuries among the highest of any occupation. The most basic of workers' rights are violated, and it is well documented that psychological and emotional trauma, as well as symptoms of Post-Traumatic Stress Disorder (PTSD), result in higher rates of domestic assault, drug, and alcohol abuse (Perussello, 2022).

The evidence is clear that our reliance on animals as a food source has brought harm on so many levels, from the innocent animals exploited and killed, to the global disease burden, food insecurity, resource overuse, and environmental depletion. A global shift to plant-based eating is an important step toward compassionate living that will bring us into greater harmonious alignment with the planet. Notably, an extensive 2023 study headed by Dr. Peter Scarborough at the University of Oxford points out how vegan diets can reduce climate change emissions, land use, and water pollution by 75 percent compared to meat-centric diets (Scarborough et al., 2023). Perhaps the urgent necessity to transform our global food practices is best summed up by Dr. Alex Lockwood from the University of Sunderland when he says: "If we were beginning from scratch with a fresh sheet of paper, no one would design the food system we currently have. Animals would not appear in our Western food system if the criteria were economic, environmental and health impacts alone" (Lockwood, 2021).

Chapter 2

Making the Transition to Plant-based Eating

As food production is the leading cause of animal suffering and the most consequential form of animal (ab)use, animal advocacy efforts often concentrate on plant-based eating. However, let it be clear that veganism is not a diet; it is an ethical stance against the exploitation of others. Animal farming, testing, hunting, riding, fishing, bullfighting, wool production, circuses, and zoos are all forms of animal oppression.

In this chapter, you will learn how to transition to a plant-based diet in a healthy and harmonious manner. The secret is to remember the *many* positive aspects of your decision rather than focusing on perceived restrictions. After all, becoming vegan is all about liberation and *true freedom*.

2.1 You Already Eat Plant-based Food

As you make the transition to a vegan lifestyle, the wonderful thing to realize is that you already eat many foods that *are* vegan! Take a few minutes (or longer) to jot down a list of all the plant-based food items you regularly eat and drink, and you will find yourself with a very long list; for example:

- Pasta and pasta sauces*
- Rice
- Beans
- Vegetables
- Fruits

- Nuts and seeds
- Hummus
- Nut butters and jams
- Oatmeal and cereals*
- Breads*
- Many snack foods,* such as chips, crackers, cookies, candy, and bars
- Olives, pickles, and condiments
- Juices
- Coffee and tea

*Check ingredients, as some may include animal products.

As you can see, you have already taken the initial step with all the vegan foods you already eat, and you will continue to add more and more foods as you expand and diversify your food repertoire.

Shifting your diet is just as much about your mindset and perceptions as it is about specific food and meal choices. Going vegan is not about reaching some state of perfection—an impossible task—in which you limit food choices or deprive yourself of the pleasures of eating. Rather, your plant-based path is an ongoing opportunity to create your own unique journey of exploration as you learn about and discover new sensations of taste, accompanied by the benefits of improved health and well-being.

2.2 Ways to Make the Transition

You may be asking yourself: "What is the best way to go plant-based?" The answer is that there are *many* ways to make the transition. Changes to any aspect of one's lifestyle can seem challenging, but you can take it at your own pace based on your individual needs and what is most comfortable for you. The steps taken will lead to lasting beneficial changes to your well-being, and it's about enjoying the journey; there are many right paths. Our food habits are influenced by many factors, among them health, family traditions, and economic, social, religious, and ethical concerns, so we should bring patience, openness, and flexibility to the process as we discover the many benefits of plant-based eating.

Some people may shift their diets overnight; for others, adapting to new food choices is best done gradually, step by step. Our personal motivations and how we each adapt to change are influential as well. A healthy dose of optimism is helpful, too, as well as not being judgmental toward ourselves or critical about the speed with which we adapt to dietary changes. We can remind ourselves that every plant-based meal makes a difference! Our continuing journey goes beyond aspects of food and health to the realization that a vibrant, nourishing lifestyle is possible without hurting other living beings.

While introducing healthy plant foods into the diet and decreasing or eliminating unhealthy ultra-processed foods, many vegans find their sensation of taste becomes more pronounced, with a brightening of the palate as it adjusts to an expanded range of flavors, not only of fruits and vegetables, but also whole grains, nuts, herbs, and seeds.

In the process of transitioning, a three- to six-week period is recommended to allow yourself to adapt. Not only are your tastes evolving, but your body is undergoing positive transformations at the cellular level. As gastroenterologist Dr. Shilpa Ravella notes, "We have evidence to back up the idea that even if you go a few weeks without junk foods and animal products high in salt, fat, and sugar, your tastes start to change" (Ravella, 2022).

It is not uncommon for newcomers to veganism to experience a few symptoms in the beginning months as the body's digestive system adjusts to the reduced intake of animal products and greater consumption of carbohydrates, especially fiber. A rapid and substantial rise in fiber intake can result in increased gas and bloating, but in most cases this subsides after a couple of weeks as your gut adjusts. Introducing fiber more gradually, especially in the case of beans, may lessen these effects, as well as being sure to drink an adequate amount of water each day and chewing your food slowly so that salivary enzymes can work right away in breaking down food. This may also apply to raw cruciferous vegetables, such as broccoli, cabbage, and cauliflower. Soaking dried beans before cooking them is a great way of removing phytic acid and carbohydrates that cause bloating. If you are using canned beans, rinsing them well will help remove the complex sugars that can cause flatulence and reduce the sodium often added to canned products. Some find that taking an enzyme supplement such as Bean-zyme® is helpful as well.

In making their dietary shift, some vegans will occasionally consume too little food and thus fewer calories, leading to feelings of low energy. This can be remedied by including high-calorie foods in the diet, such as sweet potatoes, avocados, nuts and nut butters, seeds, quinoa, tahini, tempeh, coconut products, and dried fruits.

Although not a common symptom, headaches could be related to any number of issues, including inadequate levels of hydration, vitamin D, vitamin B12, or magnesium, as well as food withdrawal symptoms. In actuality, a vegan diet has often been found to alleviate chronic headaches and migraines (Bunner et al., 2014).

While not present in all cases, physical and psychological symptoms accompanying the change in diet, including food cravings, should not be altogether surprising. This is essentially a reshaping of one's physiology and, for many, overcoming a lifetime of acquired ingrained food habits based on the consumption of animals and their products. Plant-based eating is not as much a detoxification as it is about allowing the body to come into balance at its optimal level. It boosts the gut microbiome, the trillions of microorganisms in our bodies responsible for regulating metabolism and the immune system. By regularly eating a diversity of plant-based foods, we sustain our natural abilities to heal, ward off diseases, and function with increased energy and vitality.

So, what are some specific strategies for going plant-based? Again, there is no acknowledged "best" way. And it is not necessarily a predictable path, as you will continually discover new foods and ingredients, find recipes that you like (and *don't* like), test out many new dishes, and navigate the social challenges that may arise in your interactions with others. Remember, this is not a contest, but an exciting opportunity to see food in a new light, a way to improve health, and grow and expand mental, emotional, and spiritual capacities in ways unique to *your* life! Remind yourself that the more you move toward a WFPB diet, the sooner you will begin reaping its many rewards. Here, we suggest three broad steps: 1) setting the stage, 2) a two-week exploration of plant meals, and 3) becoming fully plant-based in another month.

Setting the Stage

As with any new endeavor, especially one directly impacting your life and well-being, it is beneficial to begin by setting a foundation and acquiring basic knowledge that will be key to moving forward as you embrace the plant-based lifestyle.

1. Become familiar with the basics of what veganism is all about. In this day and age, there is a plethora of information in the form of books, websites, podcasts, blogs, online interviews, and documentaries. Vegfests have popped up in most major cities, and social media groups and in-person meetups provide information about plant-based living, offer valuable support, and allow you to interact with others and make new like-minded friends. The end of Chapter 7 includes a helpful list of resources. It contains programs with tips and guidance on going vegan, such as Challenge 22 and the Physicians Committee for Responsible Medicine (PCRM) 21-Day Vegan Kickstart Program and Vegan Starter Kit.

2. Each of us has unique life experiences that influence our food choices, and self-reflection is a wonderful way to create a deeper awareness of our personal values and motivations. Ask yourself questions such as the following:

   - Why do I want to go vegan?
   - What benefits do I hope to gain?
   - What are some aspects of my current diet that I wish to change?
   - Are there other facets of my lifestyle that I wish to improve?
   - What challenges might I expect in going plant-based?

   Throughout your vegan journey, you can periodically circle back to these questions and assess your progress. Many find that the shifting of food habits and behaviors not only results in improved health, but also opens up possibilities for greater mental clarity, new attitudes and outlooks, and even elevated spiritual awareness. Our values, motivations, and sense of self naturally go through changes, and adopting plant-based eating can bring about unexpected benefits and personal transformation.

3. An excellent, practical way to track your successes and make plant-based eating easy to implement is by putting together your own personalized vegan recipe journal. This can be a physical notebook for compiling recipes, or a digital version. It can include the following:

- Copies of your favorite recipes, organized in categories as follows:
    - Breakfast
    - Lunch
    - Dinner
    - Sides
    - Salads
    - Soups
    - Snacks and appetizers
    - Sauces, dips, dressings, and condiments
    - Desserts
    - Breads
    - Plant-based alternatives (as an example, for eggs)
    - Beverages

Before you know it, you will have a very large repertoire of meal ideas and options, always at hand to choose from and use in creating shopping lists.
- A health section, should you want to note physical changes, weight, medical test results, or other tips and information on nutrition
- A personal journal section in which you jot down thoughts and observations about any aspects of your vegan journey
- If you attend many conferences, vegfests, or online events, you can even consider a separate notebook to write down new ideas and helpful information. Once you are plant-based, you will find there is always more to learn and discover!

Begin: A Two-week Exploration of Plant-based Dishes

As we are comfortable with the foods we already eat and often have a long history with them, this is a great place to start. Beginning with familiar dishes makes adjusting to vegan versions easy with almost no extra effort, dispelling the myth that going plant-based requires a total overhaul of your cooking skills. Keep in mind that moving toward plant-based eating is never about deprivation or missing out on delicious food; rather, it is a widening of taste and flavor possibilities as you discover the extraordinary range of ingredients and meals that help to maintain your body at its best. Starting with a two-week exploration is a good way to "get your feet wet" and see how easy it is to go vegan!

During these two weeks, make it a goal to come up with twelve different main dishes that you like, covering breakfast, lunch, and dinner. For example, you may come up with three for breakfast, four for lunch, and five for dinner. These can be added to your journal.

These are three basic ways to start gathering your vegan recipes:

1. First, an easy practical step is to jot down dishes you currently eat that are *already* vegan! Add these to the recipe list in your logbook and note if there are any ways you can improve on them. As an example, let's say you regularly use pre-packaged servings of oatmeal plus dried fruit. Typically, there is not much in the way of actual fruit (though the picture on the package often suggests otherwise), and sugar and salt are usually added. Keeping in mind that the goal is to eat healthy WFPB options, it is just as easy to buy a large container of organic quick-rolled oats (with nothing added), add in fresh fruit, nuts, ground flax and/or chia seeds, and even mix in a small amount of nut butter. This not only improves the nutritive value of your meal, but also adds a diversity of healthy ingredients; it is also much more economical.

2. Next, one of the easiest things to do is what has become known as "veganizing," taking one of your favorite dishes and using simple substitutions to make it vegan. These "new" recipes can be added to your growing list of meal options.

It couldn't be easier! Google the name of a dish followed by "veganize," and numerous recipe options will pop up. For example, chickpeas can substitute for fish in a tuna sandwich; seitan can take the place of chicken in stir-frying; beans, lentils, tofu, seitan, jackfruit, seeds, and nuts—all these and more can take the place of meat. In your recipe search, note that some will use meat alternatives. These popular plant-based products have seen a phenomenal rise in the food business landscape and are found in just about all mainstream grocery stores. While these products can be used as transition foods to veganism, *some* are highly processed and thus high in salt, refined oils, and calories. Ultimately, the goal should be to minimize the use of unhealthy processed foods in favor of whole foods as close to their natural state as possible.

3. This is where the fun comes in. With all the terrific vegan websites, cookbooks, and literally thousands of vegan recipes on the internet, select and try a few brand-new recipes. Hint: choose some of your favorite foods and do a search. For example, type in "broccoli," "pasta," "easy," "vegan," and "dinner," and dozens of recipes will come up. You can also narrow down the search with modifiers such as "no oil," "sugar-free," or "gluten-free." Don't be afraid to try new dishes; be adventurous! It's fine if a dish doesn't turn out; we have all had the experience where a recipe (vegan or not) simply isn't to our satisfaction and not what we expected, and any professional chef will tell you that trial and error is all a part of the process.

Next: Fully Plant-based in 28 Days

Now that you have a number of recipes under your belt, use the next four weeks to fully transition to eating plant-based. As mentioned before, everyone goes at their own pace, but four weeks is an ideal length of time to put your new eating and shopping habits in place. We all have busy schedules with the demands and pressures of everyday life, so it is wise to be realistic about setting your goals. Some of you may find that going plant-based over a month works well. Others may want to make the transition more quickly, perhaps even going vegan overnight! The guidelines provided here are suggested as a general outline to assist you in implementing your own personal plan. Regardless of exactly how you do it, going plant-based is one of the most transformative and meaningful lifestyle steps you can take, and it will have lasting positive impacts on the rest of your life.

This is one suggested plan for each of the weeks:

- Week 1—Make all of your *breakfast* meals plant-based
- Week 2—In addition to breakfasts, make all *lunches* plant-based
- Week 3—Continue by adding plant-based *dinner* meals every day
- Week 4—You have now reached the point where *all* your meals will be vegan!

While you may have repeated some of these meals during the past few weeks (for many people, this will be the case with breakfasts and certainly with leftovers), this week could be a time to explore fruits, vegetables, food items, and ingredients that are new to you. These might include quinoa, buckwheat, farro, tempeh, tofu, seaweed, and produce you may not have tried before, such as jicama, jackfruit, dragon fruit, kohlrabi, and taro root. These are just a few of the many foods that make up the rainbow of plant-based eating.

Another variation of the four-week plan is to use days of the week as your framework. For example:

- Week 1—Make all your meals plant-based on two days (for example, Sunday and Monday)
- Week 2—In addition to those two days, add two more days (Tuesday and Wednesday)
- Week 3—Add two more days (Thursday and Friday)
- Week 4—Add in the final day (Saturday)

Naturally, you may come up with a different plan, but the goal is to create a framework so that you are eating *all* plant-based meals by the end of the four-week period. This should include any snacks as well. As you accumulate recipes, compile them in your journal, and you will have created a large collection of plant-based meals that gives you a solid foundation for continuing your vegan journey.

As you move through the twenty-eight day transition period, you may occassionally feel like eating out or meeting others for a meal. Opt for establishments that use fresh, organic whole foods. The obvious advantage of food prepataion at home is knowing exactly what ingredients are going into everything you make. Unhealthy restaurant food often uses processed oils and extra salt and sugar, products you generally want to avoid on a WFPB diet. There is also the issue of cross-contamination, which may happen if vegan foods are prepared with the same equipment used for non-vegan food, or ingredients accidentally get mixed in the same preparation area.

Overall, direct any concerns about food ingredients or preparation to the restaurant staff. This gives you a unique opportunity to raise awareness about veganism. Servers, for example, probably do not know enough about the specific ingredients in a particular dish, and you can request that they check with the chef. Animal products are often "hidden" in sauces, such as butter, honey, eggs, beef stock in the tomato sauce of a veggie pizza, or the fish and oyster sauces frequently used in Asian dishes. As a consumer paying for food at a price undoubtedly more expensive than if you prepared the dish yourself, knowing the ingredients in the dishes you order is in your interest.

Once you have shifted to plant-based eating, take a moment to reflect on what you are experiencing—changes you may have started noticing with health and well-being, your energy levels, as well as any feelings, thoughts, or personal discoveries. Food is not only a source of physical nourishment—it feeds the energy that shapes our lives every single day.

2.3 Types of Plant-based Diets, With a Focus on a Whole Food Plant-based Diet

Plant-based diets are those that include foods and beverages made from plants, fungi, and algae, and exclude all types of animal-derived products. However, not all plant-based diets are the same, as they can prioritize different aspects. For example, a diet based on raw plant foods significantly differs from one that relies on large amounts of meat and dairy analogues replicating the Western way of eating. Although both respect the ethical principle of not using animals, their nutritional value, environmental footprint, and cost vary. Here are some common types of plant-based diets:

WFPB: Focuses on minimally processed plant foods, such as fruits, vegetables, whole grains, legumes, nuts, and seeds, as well as mushrooms and algae. It limits or excludes junk food, refined sugars, and sometimes oils.

Raw vegan: Consists of uncooked, unprocessed plant foods, such as fruits, vegetables, nuts, and seeds. Cooking is typically limited to temperatures below 48°C (118°F) to preserve nutrients.

Raw till 4: A variation of the raw vegan diet where individuals eat raw, plant-based foods until 4 p.m. and may include a cooked plant-based meal in the evening.

Fruitarian: Consists primarily of fruits, with some variations allowing for seeds, nuts, and certain plant-based foods. The restrictive nature of fruitarianism can make it challenging to meet essential nutrient requirements, and it may not be suitable for everyone. This is especially true in parts of the world where fruit is not produced in abundance due to climate restraints.

Gluten-free vegan: A variation of the WFPB diet, where foods and beverages containing a protein called gluten are excluded. In practice, this means excluding products made of wheat, barley, rye, triticale, and other grains containing gluten. It is important to note that there are many naturally gluten-free foods, such as fruits, vegetables, beans, lentils, nuts, seeds, and gluten-free grains like rice, quinoa, and corn. Additionally, there is an increasing availability of gluten-free alternatives for many traditionally gluten-containing products.

These plant-based diets offer different approaches to incorporating plant foods into one's eating habits. Most people eating plant-based follow a WFPB diet or a variation, with a large portion of whole plant foods and small amounts of sugar and market-bought dairy and meat alternatives. A slice of cake now and then does not hurt anyone!

Individuals may choose the plant-based diet that best aligns with their health goals, ethical considerations, and personal preferences. It is important to note that a well-balanced plant-based diet should provide adequate nutrients, and individuals may benefit from consulting with a healthcare professional or a registered dietitian specializing in plant-based nutrition for personalized guidance.

In this book, we focus on the WFPB diet, which has been proven time and time again to offer multiple health benefits. This diet is also highly varied and convenient given the abundance of the plant, algae, and fungi kingdoms. We already discussed the health effects of transitioning to plant-based eating in Chapter 1 (section 1.2), but here is a summary of the top ten potential health benefits of a WFPB diet:

1. **Healthier heart**: The nutrient content of the WFPB diet can lower blood pressure and serum cholesterol, reducing the risk of cardiovascular conditions like heart disease, stroke, and vascular cognitive impairment (VCI) (Wang et al., 2023).

2. **Improved digestion and metabolism**: A higher intake of fiber and essential nutrients in a WFPB diet prevents constipation, reduces chronic inflammation, and promotes a balanced gut microbiota, potentially lowering the risk of many conditions, from obesity to bowel disorders to cancer (Matsushita et al., 2023).

3. **Diabetes prevention and control**: The elimination of risk factors present in animal products along with the nutrient content of a WFPB diet balances insulin secretion and blood sugar levels, helping prevent, manage, and even reverse type 2 diabetes (Wang et al., 2023; Thomas et al., 2023).

4. **Reduced body inflammation**: The nutrients in a WFPB diet promote antioxidant defences that reduce inflammation, oxidative stress, and hormonal imbalance, lowering the risk and severity of a range of health conditions, such as acne, psoriasis, PCOS, obesity, and cancer (Fusano, 2023; Chavez et al., 2023).

5. **Lower cancer risk**: Limited exposure to cancer-promoting substances often found in animal products combined with the nutrients provided by the WFPB diet can lower the risk of cancer, especially digestive cancer and breast cancer (WHO & IARC, 2015; Dunneram et al., 2019; DeClercq et al., 2022; Melnik et al., 2023; Guéraud et al., 2024).

6. **Kidney disease prevention and mitigation**: Blood pressure regulation, reduced protein intake, and higher intake of antioxidant compounds provided by a WFPB diet help protect the kidneys and control the progression of kidney conditions (Zarantonello & Brunori, 2023).

7. **Hormonal balance and fertility**: The nutrient content of a WFPB diet and the absence of animal hormones may modulate hormone levels, insulin secretion, and sensitivity, contributing to better metabolic health, overall fertility, and a lower risk of hormone-related conditions, from acne to POS to cancer (Wang et al., 2023; Łakoma et al., 2023).

8. **Women's health and men's health**: In women, a balanced plant-based diet may mitigate symptoms linked to PMS, PCOS, and menopause, including menstrual cramps, mood swings, bloating, and hot flashes (Barnard, 2020). A WFPB diet may also reduce the risk of female cancer, including breast and endometrial cancer (Dunneram et al., 2019). In men, a WFBP may lower the risk of prostate cancer (Matsushita et al., 2023).

9. **Healthier brain**: Healthy plant-based diets protect against cognitive decline through the increased intake of antioxidants and poly-unsaturated fats and the lower intake of inflammatory compounds, reducing the risk of Alzheimer's disease and VCI (Ding et al., 2022).

10. **Better immunity and longevity**: Evidence suggests that people who follow a WFPB diet live longer and healthier. This may be attributed to the nutrient content and lower exposure to toxins, cholesterol, saturated fats, and animal hormones, leading to a range of health benefits (Herpich et al., 2022; Wang et al., 2023; Thomas et al., 2023). Positive habits and outlooks on life commonly found among vegans, such as respect for life, meditation, and physical activity, are additional factors leading to improved mental and physical health.

Of course, while a WFPB diet offers many health benefits, individual responses can vary. Additionally, proper planning is crucial to ensure that your diet provides essential nutrients, including calcium, vitamin B12, iron, and omega-3 fatty acids. Consulting with a healthcare professional or registered dietitian trained in plant-based nutrition can help individuals tailor a balanced diet to their health needs and goals.

2.4 Making Your Meals Plant-based

Everyone eats plants, so transitioning to a plant-based diet involves incorporating more plant foods while reducing animal products. While this can be done either gradually or overnight, your body may need time to adapt to new habits. Here are some practical tips to make your meals plant-based.

Start gradually: Begin by gradually increasing the proportion of plant foods in your meals. You can start with one plant-based meal per day and gradually expand from there. It can be helpful to set a time goal, for example: "I will be 100 percent plant-based within four weeks." Need extra motivation? Think of the animals!

Explore plant proteins: Incorporate plant-based protein sources into your meals, such as beans, lentils, chickpeas, tofu, tempeh, edamame, and plant-based meat alternatives. They help with nutrition and satiety and can be used to replicate flavors, textures, and appearances associated with animal products.

Swap animal-origin products with plant-based substitutes: Replace eggs, dairy, meat, and fish with plant-based equivalents. For example, order an oat cappuccino instead of a dairy cappuccino, choose a bean burrito over a beef burrito, and replace chicken with tempeh pieces in your Caesar salad.

Experiment with whole grains: Choose brown rice, quinoa, barley, oats, and whole wheat instead of refined grains. Whole grains provide fiber and essential nutrients, in addition to ensuring more satiety in fewer kilocalories.

Include a variety of vegetables: Aim to fill half of your plate with vegetables. Include a colorful mix of leafy greens, bell peppers, tomatoes, carrots, and more.

Add fruits: Incorporate fresh fruits into your meals or have them as snacks. They can add natural sweetness and a variety of nutrients to your diet. Starting your day with oatmeal, granola, or a smoothie packed with fresh fruit is an easy way to increase your daily fruit intake.

Embrace nuts and seeds: Include nuts and seeds in your meals for healthy fats (including omega-3) and additional protein. Sprinkle them on salads, oatmeal, or yogurt.

Explore plant-based dairy alternatives: Try plant-based milk alternatives like almond, soy, coconut, oat milk, and others. Try them all and discover your favorite. You will notice that some are perfect for sweet recipes, while others are great to drink from the glass. Additionally, experiment with plant-based cheeses, yogurts, and other dairy substitutes.

Use plant-based oils: Choose plant-based oils such as olive oil and canola oil for cooking and dressings. They provide essential fatty acids with little to no saturated fats, unlike coconut oil, which has a higher fraction of saturated fats. While certainly healthier than animal fats, plant oils are best used sparingly, as they are calorically dense (1 tablespoon of olive oil contains over 100 calories!), with no fiber (Greger, 2015).

Utilize herbs and spices: Enhance the flavor of your meals with herbs and spices. Experiment with different combinations to add variety and depth to your dishes. This is an excellent way to reduce your salt intake.

Learn new recipes: Explore plant-based recipes to find inspiration. Countless delicious and creative plant-based dishes are available online and in plant-based cookbooks. You can also adapt traditional recipes by using plant-based alternatives to animal-origin ingredients. Check section 2.5 for more details.

Meal prep and planning: Plan your meals ahead of time and consider batch cooking. Having plant-based meals readily available can make it easier to stick to your dietary goals.

Educate yourself: We have been bombarded with propaganda and misinformation on diet and health since childhood, so learn about plant-based nutrition from *reliable* sources to ensure you are getting a well-balanced diet.

Connect with the plant-based community: Join online forums, social media groups, or local communities that focus on plant-based living. You can gain support, share experiences, and discover new recipes.

Know why you are doing it: There are many crucial reasons to become plant-based, including animal rights, human rights, health, environmental sustainability, and the contribution to a nonviolent world. Keep these reasons in mind and be confident that you are doing the right thing for you and everyone else.

As previously mentioned, people may complain of feeling gassy when they first become plant-based. This is a common symptom that will disappear with time—unless you have a medical condition, like irritable bowel syndrome (IBS), or are allergic to specific foods. By all means, avoid foods and beverages to which you are sensitive or allergic. Increased flatulence or bloating in the transition to plant-based eating is frequently associated with a higher fiber intake and the development of a more balanced gut microbiota. Do not worry; your body will eventually adjust to the new diet.

Remember that everyone's journey to a plant-based diet is unique, so find an approach that works for you. Gradual changes and experimentation with new foods will help you discover a variety of delicious and nutritious plant-based meals while giving proper time for your mind, body, and heart to adjust to a beautiful new lifestyle.

2.5 Plant-based Alternatives to Everyday Ingredients

Many traditional ingredients used in different parts of the world come from animals. Luckily, we do not need these ingredients to be happy and healthy—quite the opposite. Replacing ingredients of animal origin has never been easier. The following is a list of popular plant-based alternatives to render your meals completely animal-free.

Milk: In theory, any seed, nut, or cereal and even some fruits can be made into plant-based milk. You can find them in grocery stores or make them at home. Here are some examples:

- Soy milk
- Almond milk
- Oat milk
- Coconut milk
- Rice milk
- Homemade plant-based milk—The preparation method may differ depending on the main ingredient, but generally consists of blending it in a processor with water and filtering the mixture with a cheesecloth. Hard ingredients (such as nuts, seeds, and rice) can be soaked beforehand for a smoother texture after blending. There are also many excellent milk maker machines on the market.

Butter: Dairy butter can be replaced with different ingredients, depending on the intended use. For example:
- Vegan butter
- Dairy-free margarine
- Coconut oil
- Olive oil

Condensed milk: An ingredient frequently used in many countries for desserts, plant-based condensed milk can be bought at the supermarket or made at home using everyday staples.
- Vegan condensed milk—Different products vary in composition, with typical options made primarily from water, sugar, and plant ingredients like oats, coconut, or soybeans. There are many brands to choose from nowadays.
- Homemade plant-based condensed milk—Broadly speaking, making condensed milk involves cooking a blend of sugar and milk until a thick consistency is achieved.

Evaporated milk: Just like condensed milk, you can find evaporated milk in the supermarket or make it at home. The process is easier than the one for condensed milk, as it involves a single ingredient: the plant milk of our choice.
- Vegan evaporated milk
- Homemade plant-based evaporated milk—In principle, any plant milk can be evaporated to the desired consistency, but thicker milks (like soy) will give a richer texture.

Custard: Animal-free alternatives to custard can be store-bought or homemade. Plant-based custard can be used in various desserts, such as fruit tarts, puddings, or as a topping for cakes.
- Vegan custard

- Homemade plant-based custard—Creating a plant-based custard at home is quite straightforward, and you can use your favorite plant milk to achieve a creamy and tasty result. There are many recipes online.

Yogurt: There are increasingly more plant-based yogurt options, including plain, Greek-style, and fruit-flavored yogurt. Here are some common alternatives to dairy yogurt:
- Coconut yogurt
- Almond yogurt
- Soy yogurt

Cheese: The first plant-based cheeses on the market were a blend of starch and vegetable oil that looked and even melted like the original product but did not offer the same taste. Research and development of dairy alternatives is evolving rapidly, and realistic cultured cheese is increasingly available. Whether you are looking for hard cheese to be consumed on its own, grated cheese for pizza, or spreadable cheese, there are options for every taste:
- Cashew cheese
- Almond cheese
- Soy-based cheeses
- Nutritional yeast—This superfood makes a great topping for pasta and popcorn and adds a delicious cheesy flavor to dishes and sauces.

Sour cream: Plant-based sour cream can be bought at grocery stores or prepared at home. Here are some options:
- Vegan sour cream—There are different brands to choose from, like Follow Your Heart, Only Plant Based!, and Miyoko's.
- Homemade cashew cream—An excellent sour cream substitute is made of cashew nuts, water, olive oil, lemon juice, and nutritional yeast. Adjust the amount of lemon juice for the ideal zesty flavor. There are many recipes online.

Eggs: Eggs can be swapped with various plant-based ingredients, based on the intended use. These alternatives are not only ethical, but also cholesterol free.
- Aquafaba—The liquid from the cooking of chickpeas is called aquafaba. Its composition gives it a very similar consistency to egg whites. Aquafaba can be whipped into a foam to create a light and fluffy texture. The water from the can of chickpeas can also be used directly in both savory and sweet recipes.
- Applesauce—This can be used as a binding agent in baking.
- Mashed bananas—This can be used as a binder in sweet recipes.
- Tofu—You can make an omelette using tofu, the famous scrambled tofu. There are many delicious recipes online.
- Flaxseed or chia seed gel—Blend seeds with warm water in a processor until they form a gel that can be used in various recipes for gelling and binding effects. If you choose milled flaxseeds, there is no need to use a processor; simply blend them with warm water and let them soak for a few minutes.

Meat (red and white): Whether you are looking for whole food alternatives to meat (e.g., tofu and beans) or meat substitutes (e.g., Beyond Meat), there are abundant options that will satisfy your taste buds without hurting anyone. Please bear in mind that *traditional* meat products undergo various processing stages before reaching the consumer table, so be mindful of the misinformation claiming that animal flesh is preferable to plant-based meat because it requires less processing. There are many inaccuracies in this statement (check section 3.3 for more details). As demonstrated by robust evidence, plant-based meat alternatives are healthier than what they replace. Whole plant ingredients are, of course, even better. Here are some options:
- Tofu
- Tempeh
- Seitan
- Lentils
- Chickpeas

- Beans
- Jackfruit—This fruit is a great option to replicate the texture and mouthfeel of shredded meat.
- Banana peels—They can be used similarly to jackfruit to mimic pulled pork.
- Plant-based burgers, sausages, bacon, ham, chicken, and others—There are many styles and brands to choose from, such as Quorn, Beyond Meat, Impossible Burger, Gardein, and Linda McCartney, to name some.

Honey: Who needs to exploit the hard labor of beautiful bees in this day and age? There are natural ingredients that offer very similar taste and function:
- Maple syrup
- Date syrup

Gelatin: Gelatin can be replaced with plant- and algae-based ingredients, such as the following:
- Agar-agar (derived from seaweed)
- Carrageenan (another seaweed-based option)
- Vegan gelatin alternatives (made from agar-agar, carrageenan, and other animal-free materials)

Seafood: Fish and other aquatic animals, sadly called "seafood," can be swapped for a variety of plant- and algae-based alternatives. The texture and flavor can be made more like traditional seafood by using different cooking methods and seasonings.
- Jackfruit—This fruit has a fibrous texture that can be used to create alternatives to shredded or flaked fish in dishes like tacos or wraps.
- Hearts of palm—This delicious vegetable has a texture similar to that of crab or lobster meat, making it a popular choice for plant-based seafood alternatives, such as crab cakes or ceviche.
- Tempeh and tofu—These ingredients, which have been used for centuries in Asian countries, can be marinated and used in various seafood-inspired dishes. Both plain and smoked tofu can be cubed and stir-fried to resemble

scallops or used in sushi, while tempeh can be used for a firmer texture in dishes like fish tacos.
- Vegan fish fillets—Brands like Gardein, Good Catch, and Sophie's Kitchen offer plant-based fish fillets made from ingredients like soy, pea protein, and seaweed.
- Vegan shrimp—Companies like New Wave Foods and Sophie's Kitchen produce plant-based shrimp made from ingredients such as konjac, pea protein, and tapioca starch.
- Vegan crab cakes—Look for plant-based crab cakes made from ingredients like hearts of palm, artichokes, or jackfruit.
- Seaweed and algae products—Seaweed and algae are used to create plant-based alternatives that mimic the texture and flavor of fish, including caviar and vegan fish sauce.
- Plant-based tuna—Brands like Good Catch and Loma Linda offer plant-based tuna alternatives made from a blend of legumes and algae.
- Plant-based scallops—Some companies offer plant-based scallop alternatives made from ingredients like king oyster mushrooms or konjac.

Fish sauce: Fishes taste how they taste because they eat algae. Therefore, the best way to reproduce the taste of fish sauce is to use algae in the recipe. Here are some options:
- Algae-based spice mix
- Spirulina, dulse, wakame, kombu, and other seaweeds
- Soy sauce
- Tamari
- Coconut aminos—This is a fermented sauce made from the nectar of coconut palm flowers and sea salt.

Mayonnaise: Eggs are frequently used in mayonnaise to help bind the ingredients. But we do not need to hurt birds for the perfect mayo, spread, or dip. The following are some options that are both delicious and healthier than traditional mayo. However, one should remember that spreads and dips should be consumed sparingly as they can be high in fat and sodium, even if plant-based:

- Vegan mayonnaise—In commercial products, eggs are replaced with ingredients such as neutral-flavored oils (like canola, safflower, or sunflower), vinegar, lemon juice, aquafaba, and silken tofu for cholesterol-free mayo. You can also make it at home.
- Avocado—This fruit can be made into a spread, rich in good fats and essential fatty acids.
- Hummus and other legume-based spreads—These are delicious, protein-rich spreads.
- Pesto—Plant-based pesto is made from nuts, olive oil, greens, and herbs, such as basil, garlic, and parsley.
- Vegetable spreads—Eggplant, tomatoes, cucumber, peppers, and beetroot can be made into tasty and healthy spreads.
- Cashew sauce—Sauces made of cashew nuts, water, salt, and olive oil are tasty alternatives to mayo. Add some spoons of nutritional yeast for a cheesy flavor, vitamin B12, and extra protein. Many recipes are available online.

Cream: Dairy cream is derived from the higher-fat layer skimmed from the top of cow's milk. This product, packed with saturated fats and cholesterol, is used for cooking, topping, and baking. While the following plant-based options are still rich in fats, they are composed of mono- and polyunsaturated fats, with a much lower saturated fat content and zero cholesterol:
- Coconut cream
- Cashew cream

Worcestershire sauce: This sauce is commonly used with steaks, hamburgers, and other dishes. It is not vegan because it frequently contains anchovies. Here are some animal-free alternatives:
- Vegan Worcestershire sauce—In store-bought products, fishes are replaced with other condiments. There are also online recipes.
- Soy sauce (shoyu)—This is a fermented sauce made from soybeans, wheat, water, and salt.
- Tamari—This wheat-free sauce is made from fermented soybeans.

Meat/bone broth: Who would want to use water in which animal body parts have been boiled? Vegetables and mushrooms are great alternatives that are both tasty and rich in antioxidants. You can also use food scraps to make your own vegetable broth, including the stems and leaves of vegetables and herbs. It is easy and much cheaper than buying broth at the grocery store.
- Vegetable broth
- Mushroom broth

While this is not an exhaustive list, these alternatives demonstrate the endless options we have available for plant-based cooking. Many can be easily made at home using a single ingredient (e.g., oat milk), while others involve a blend of ingredients commonly used for home cooking (e.g., cashew sour cream). For extra convenience, many of these alternatives are found in the supermarket. Keep in mind that the availability of these products may vary depending on your location, and new plant-based alternatives are continually being developed.

2.6 How to Navigate Social Challenges

Going plant-based is a transition to new ways of healthy eating, but it also comes with particular challenges with regard to social situations. This is true not only for new vegans, but longtime ones as well. Sometimes this can be a source of stress, as many social activities and interactions often revolve around food. Vegans experience a wide range of reactions, from those non-vegans who are supportive and open to understanding why we make the dietary choices we do, to those who may be confrontational or hostile, even engaging in ridicule. This can be especially difficult, as it is natural for us to want our close family and friends to be open to the lifestyle choices that are so important and meaningful to us.

As in other aspects of our relationships, engaging with others about veganism is most positive when we take into account their unique personalities and where they are coming from. How we interact with one person may be totally different from how we do so with another. We have likely acquired much information about plant-based eating and its numerous benefits, and many of us are eager to share what we know. At the same time, it is helpful to keep in mind that for many people, the idea of veganism has not even occurred to them. Our interactions with them may very well be the very first time they have met a vegan! We can see this as a positive step in that our engagement with them is already planting a seed of awareness that a healthier and more compassionate lifestyle actually exists.

These are some general guidelines for navigating social settings as a vegan:

1. Focus on keeping the interaction as you would any other conversation—being assertive but also open, receptive, and positive. Unfortunately, there exists a stereotype of the "self-righteous" vegan, which serves as a means to deflect attention from the harm inflicted on animals. As animal advocates, we certainly wish that everyone we meet would become vegan, but our communication with others will be most productive by just being our normal, relaxed selves and remembering that most of us were once in their shoes! In that way, they will be more open to what we say without feeling they are being judged or criticized, and we can keep the focus on advocating for the animals. Obviously, there are times, places, and events to be more upfront in promoting animal rights, but social, personal conversations may call for a different approach. It is not necessarily a question of whether to speak up or not, but rather gauging the audience and context to choose the right strategy and tone. Frequently, waiting for an opportune moment to express one's views may yield more positive outcomes in the long run. With time, you will learn how to read the situation.

2. Part of the challenge in social settings is that some non-vegans may, perhaps on a subconscious level, feel judged or threatened just by the fact that you are vegan and they are not. This can trigger a type of fight-or-flight response where they feel defensive, even though at a deep level they are probably aware of the cruelty connected with using animals. Keeping our communications positive and speaking from the place of compassion that we all share will help the other person to be accepting of us and open to understanding what veganism is all about.

3. It is always helpful to point out, to the degree that is compatible with the given situation, how being vegan has helped *you*. We should never underestimate how much we can inspire others just by being positive models for plant-based living. Many vegans can probably point out common questions they receive, such as, "How do you stay so healthy?" or "Where do you get all your energy?" Vegan psychologist Clare Mann puts it best when she says, "The best thing a vegan can do is to be a great example of a happy, adjusted, open-minded, caring person who also happens to be vegan" (Mann, 2018).

4. While we understandably would like the whole world to go vegan right away, it is helpful to take a step back and remember our *own* personal history when we were pre-vegan. Most of us grew up in a culture with the ingrained acceptance of using animals, and there is strong inertia to maintain longtime habits, no matter how consequential they are. Remind yourself that people of integrity do exist, and many may only be "asleep" (like we were when we used to harm animals ourselves). We can maintain a healthy perspective by embracing the positive qualities we see in all others, whether or not they are vegan.

5. Take the time to educate yourself about all things vegan. The more informed you are, the better you will be able to share knowledge with clarity and confidence. You will also be able to address some of the most common misconceptions that come up.

Here are some of the most common scenarios you may encounter, along with advice and strategies:

You are invited to a meal or gathering at someone's home, where the hosts do not realize you are vegan.

Contact the host ahead of time to let them know you are vegan. They may include a vegan dish in their planning, but you can offer to bring along a vegan dish or dishes.

You are invited to a potluck or social gathering.

This is a wonderful opportunity to show how delicious it is to eat plant-based! Note: Sometimes people can be turned off knowing beforehand that a dish is vegan. (Yes, people are conditioned to the point they are grossed out by plants and not by body parts and fluids on their plate!) One strategy is not mentioning that the dish you brought is vegan. Then, when you start receiving compliments, say something like, "Oh, by the way, that's plant-based!" Guests will be impressed and more open to how easy and amazing it can be to eat as a vegan.

You are meeting friends at a restaurant that is not all-vegan.

More and more restaurants now offer vegan options. Check out the menu online ahead of time and see what the possibilities are, or even call to find out more information. For example, if in an Italian restaurant, ask if their tomato sauce is vegan. Or with Asian restaurants, check to see if fish sauce is used. Note that you will likely encounter restaurant staff who do not fully understand what *vegan* means. This actually gives us a unique opportunity to educate others about ingredients in vegan foods.

You are discussing restaurant options with friends.

By becoming familiar with area restaurants with vegan options, you could suggest these as possibilities to your friends.

You are attending a reception or conference where meals will be served.

It pays to check in advance. More and more event planners are aware of people with special-needs diets, whether vegetarian, vegan, gluten-free, and so on. Once on-site, mention to the kitchen staff or servers that you have arranged for a vegan meal.

Non-vegan guests or family are visiting your home for a few days.

It is important to let them know *ahead of time* that you have a vegan household. This gives them the opportunity to stay elsewhere, such as a hotel or Airbnb, if they don't want to eat plant-based during the visit. Cooking for guests, however, is a chance to show how delicious vegan meals can be!

Friends or family push back on your decision to be vegan, or are outright confrontational.

It is a good idea to briefly explain the reasons for your diet change, citing a mix of reasons—for your health, how you feel about animals, and environmental concerns. Communicating this does not require a lengthy explanation. Keep it light and as positive as possible to avoid an argument or conflict. When we receive an aggressive response, it may be that they actually feel some sense of conflict within, and sometimes it is that very person who eventually decides to try going plant-based!

Someone you know is curious as to why you are vegan.

First, gauge where someone is coming from, as this will give you an indication of what and how much to say. Everyone has their own personal background, circumstances, and influences surrounding food choices and ethical stances. As in any discussion, it is important to *listen*, for communication is a two-way street. Asking questions gives us context for a productive conversation where the other person feels understood, increasing the chances that they will be more open to what we share. These situations are not about showing that you are right or winning an argument. It is about having a meaningful shared interaction so they gain some awareness and understanding of your vegan values. Asking non-vegans questions is a great way to make them notice the moral inconsistencies in their own reasoning.

Someone says, "You don't mind if I eat meat, do you?"

The nature of your response to this common question will depend a lot on the individual you are responding to, but one might reply by asking the person a question such as, "I'm curious, why did you say that?" The question could open the door to engaging with the person in a positive conversation where you feel comfortable expressing why you have chosen to be vegan. It will also give you insights into where they are coming from and to what degree they may be curious about plant-based eating. The fact that someone asks this question reflects that, on some level, they are aware that we choose not to consume animals for a good reason, and we can use this opportunity to raise their awareness.

An important family gathering is taking place, such as Thanksgiving, where turkey or other animal products will be served.

Contact the host ahead of time and let them know you can contribute to the dinner by bringing vegan dishes and even a dessert. Oftentimes, the "side" dishes are the favorite highlights of these meals. Keep in mind, above all, how blessed we are to be able to spend time with our close ones. Understandably, some will feel that it is too painful to sit down at a shared meal where a fellow animal is the centerpiece. In such cases, some vegans decide not to attend or perhaps choose to visit once the meal is completed. Whatever the case, it is important to be sensible. As your family circle permits, politely decline the invitation, expressing your reason for doing that with honesty and kindness. Healthy and assertive dialogues are a powerful way to raise awareness. Another way to get around the social difficulties of holiday meals is to create your own all-vegan dinner event!

Someone makes fun of you for being vegan.

We have all heard of the scenario where someone jokingly asks something like, "So what do you eat, salads?" In situations like this, remaining composed and keeping your response appropriate to the context will help them see that being vegan is not something extreme or baseless. You could respond with a light statement such as, "Well, there's actually many foods we eat, and they are delicious and super healthy!" This statement opens the door to a possible positive conversation. You can also smile and amicably reply with another question, such as "Why would you think that vegans only eat salad?" If the environment allows (e.g., you are talking with close friends), you may be more upfront and say something like, "I eat everything except for animal body parts and secretions." There is nothing wrong with this sentence; it is factual and thought-provoking—and it all depends on your tone.

An acquaintance reacts to your veganism with outright hostility or even bullying.

When faced with gratuitous aggressiveness in response to your veganism, it is essential to prioritize your well-being and maintain a calm and assertive demeanor.

Dialoguing with a reasonable person is one thing, but engaging in conversation with narrow-minded or ill-intentioned people is a waste of your time and energy. In such cases, for your own well-being, it may be decided to no longer connect with them. This includes in-person interactions as well as social media.

You are living with someone who is not vegan.

This scenario may arise if, for example, you are sharing a living space with a roommate or family member. Some have adapted to this situation by having specific refrigerator/freezer space for each person, as well as having a clear separation of cookware and utensils. You may on occasion cook a vegan dish to share. But ultimately, one has to assess the practicality and viability of such a situation according to their own personal values and needs. If it is simply too difficult to live in a place where animals are consumed and used, your best choice may be to seek a different living arrangement.

What if you feel alone or isolated as a beginning vegan?

In this day and age, there are so many ways to reach out and find support. These include local meet-up groups or community vegan societies, numerous social media groups, and opportunities to participate in events through Zoom to share ideas and knowledge and discuss the challenges of going vegan. Attending cooking classes, conferences, and vegfests are additional ways to engage with like-minded folks and receive extra motivation and positive feedback about the benefits of being vegan. As you expand your circle of vegan friends, spending time and meals with them is a great way to maintain a positive social outlook, as connections with them can provide a strong boost to confidence and emotional well-being.

Chapter 3

Plant-based Food Shopping Guide

3.1 Eating Plant-based is Cheaper than Eating Animal Products

A central practical question in going plant-based is how to increase the fraction of plant foods while reducing the fraction of animal foods. When vegans advocate for healthy, ethical, and eco-friendly eating, we are often accused of privilege for promoting something inaccessible to the average person. Even when genuine, this concern is unfounded. People tend to assume that a plant-based diet is expensive when we all know that meat, dairy, and fish are pricey. See Figure 5, for example.

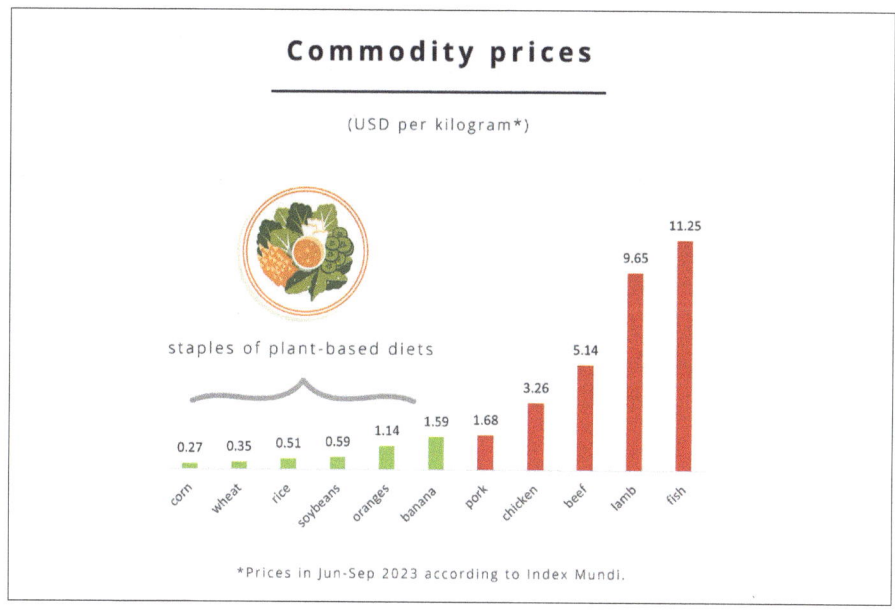

Figure 5. *Average price of food commodities globally. Data source: www.indexmundi.com/commodities/.*

In fact, studies show that eating plant foods is cheaper than eating an omnivore diet in most geographical regions (Springmann et al., 2021). We will discuss that later. But for now, let us think of *your* reality. Think of all the food items you buy every month. Now answer the following questions:

1. What are the most expensive foods in your shopping cart?
2. What are the cheapest foods in your shopping cart?
3. What percentage of your groceries are fruits, veggies, and minimally processed foods like nuts, beans, rice, and lentils?
4. How much do you spend on plant foods versus animal foods? (Think of percentages, like 50/50 or 30/70.)
5. If you replaced the meat and fish products you consume with protein-rich foods such as legumes, tofu, and tempeh, would you spend more or less on groceries?
6. Do you know how much a block of tofu or a kilogram/pound of dried beans costs and how many people it can feed?

The truth is that people are so conditioned to eating in a certain way that most of them do not even know what a WFPB diet looks like. So how could they possibly conclude that it is expensive to eat plant-based?

The average omnivore centers their diet around products like eggs, cow's milk, cheese, chicken breast, ground beef, steak, sausages, bacon, etc. That is one of the main reasons why people think of a plant-based diet as an *animal-free version of their own diets*, where animal-based products are simply replaced with plant-based analogues. As we explained in Chapter 2, that is not what a WFPB diet is. Moreover, plant-based analogues can be expensive as the sector is still in its infancy. Factors like economies of scale, established markets, and financial incentives largely benefit animal products over plant-based alternatives (Vallone & Lambin, 2023).

Do not take us wrong: Plant-based alternatives replicating animal products are useful—and healthier than what they replace. For one, they help reduce the reliance on products that inflict horrific suffering on animals. Moreover, convenience plays a big role in our busy lives. The fact that we now have a wide range of high-quality substitutes for dairy products, for instance, makes our lives easier.

And prices will likely drop with the increasing demand and larger-scale production. However, replicating a diet that is *unhealthy by default* by consuming plant-based analogues instead of introducing more whole plants will result in an unbalanced and expensive diet. Most of us must relearn how to eat for health and well-being.

A recent Oxford University study revealed that plant-centered diets are significantly cheaper than omnivore diets in high- and middle-income countries such as the United States, Canada, the United Kingdom, Australia, and across Western Europe (Springmann et al., 2021). Vegan diets are the most affordable, reducing food costs by up to 33 percent. Vegetarian diets were a close second, and flexitarian diets with limited amounts of meat and dairy were 14 percent cheaper. By contrast, pescatarian diets increased costs by up to 2 percent. The research calculated the costs of diets in 150 countries from all world regions by pairing estimates of food demand for different consumption patterns with estimates of commodity prices in different years considering food system and socioeconomic changes.

But what about lower-income countries? The Oxford study also found that in countries on the Indian subcontinent and sub-Saharan Africa, eating a healthy and sustainable diet would be up to 25 percent cheaper than a typical Western diet, but at least a third more expensive than current diets. That is understandable, as food insecurity is more frequent in lower-income nations, where diets tend to include large amounts of starchy foods while lacking essential nutrients and often calories. Moreover, research shows there are many opportunities for reducing financial barriers to healthy eating across the world, including food supply improvements and strategies to curb food waste (Rao et al., 2013).

Worthy of note is that the Oxford study did not include meat analogues, eating at restaurants, or takeout/takeaways. However, eating out is a relevant aspect of the cost of plant-based eating that people tend to overlook, whether we are talking about fine dining or fast food. It costs the same to order a beef burger or a lentil burger. The vegan lasagna and the animal-based version are the same price. And, quite frankly, the most expensive dishes at a restaurant are usually those based on meat and seafood. We see this way too often: people go to a restaurant with a mixed menu and completely ignore the vegan options. So how come they conclude that eating plant-based is more expensive? This is a crystallized opinion, not based on facts, frequently used to avoid the subject.

Of course, the price of *any* diet can vary depending on where you live and the type of products you choose, including the brand, place of origin, farming method (e.g., organic), and level of processing and convenience. The same applies to a WFPB diet.

If budget is a concern, planning meals, buying in bulk, focusing on staple foods, and reducing reliance on more-processed products can help make a plant-based diet more affordable. In the following sections, we will give you more details of what to look for when buying food to save you money and time while making the best choices for your health.

3.2 Stocking Your Plant-based Kitchen

Making the shift toward plant-based living is a wonderful opportunity to take stock (literally *and* figuratively) of all the food products in your kitchen pantry. Whether you make the change all at once or gradually, it is about redefining the role of food in your life, as you discover the incredibly wide range of nutritious plant foods and the chance to explore new tastes with every meal.

It is important to realize that, for most of us, food choices are the result of long-ingrained family habits. Change is not always easy, but starting out with a well-stocked pantry provides you with the basic ingredients that serve as a foundation for creating a variety of nourishing plant-based meals.

One of the myths surrounding veganism is that one has to buy expensive, hard-to-find ingredients, but nothing could be further from the truth! Going plant-based is not about buying unusual or expensive ingredients that need extra preparation or cooking skills. Rather, it is about *simplifying* one's approach to food, reaping the benefits of consuming plants as close to their natural state as possible. A major benefit to consumers moving toward veganism is that food staples can be found in regular grocery stores, not only in health food stores.

For so many new vegans, having a kitchen newly stocked with plant foods gives them a tremendous sense of well-being. Such ingredients will boost health and contribute to a more environmentally friendly lifestyle, and new vegans will come to understand that nourishment is not derived from cruelty inflicted upon fellow beings. The benefits also extend to a clarity and brightening of mind and spirit, as one embraces a lifestyle rooted in peace and compassion. As Lin Silvan, executive director of the Eugene Veg Education Network, notes, "Any time is a good time to become vegan. Just gather new information from reliable sources, get over any skepticism, and redirect your thinking towards the greater good. Don't be skewed by long-term habits and knee-jerk resistance. It's okay not to be perfect, as long as we allow compassion to be continuously moving us forward to making better decisions. New understandings might be scary at first, but they are powerful and unrelenting, and, yes, joyful!" (Silvan, 2021).

The following list is a general guide to get started. Your vegan kitchen pantry will not necessarily include all these items, as you can build it gradually, and its contents will naturally change over time as you discover the wonderful diversity of plant foods. At the same time, you will develop a sense of which products you use regularly. Animal products in your kitchen can be disposed of, possibly given to non-vegan friends, or donated to a local food bank. Many new vegans, especially those doing so for ethical reasons, often express feelings ranging from a sense of renewal to peace and even liberation knowing that their kitchens are now cruelty-free. In addition, of course, there is the health benefit, with all food preparation in the home focusing on the nutritional power of plants. Expanding your repertoire of delicious meal options is an exciting opportunity to learn more about food and how it is key to enhanced health and wellness, deepening your commitment to a more compassionate lifestyle.

Here are a few general tips on creating your vegan kitchen:

1. Put together a rough plan of meals for the coming week to help with shopping.
2. It is helpful to keep a magnetic notepad on the refrigerator door to quickly jot down shopping items as you think of them.
3. Have healthy snack items out and always available in the kitchen or dining area. These could include fresh fruits, nuts, dried fruits, and even healthy spices that can quickly be added to salads and main dishes.
4. It helps to be aware of when particular produce items are in season and, therefore, less expensive, or on sale.

5. Frozen fruits and vegetables are just as nutritious as buying them fresh, as most are flash-frozen at maximum ripeness. Frozen produce is especially handy for creating green smoothies. Avoid canned fruits with added sugar; look for "unsweetened" or "no sugar added" instead.
6. Whole grains, nuts, and seeds are best stored long-term in airtight containers or plastic bags in the refrigerator or freezer.

Plant-based Grocery Items
- Flour
- Whole-grain flours (wheat, quinoa, spelt, buckwheat)
- All-purpose flour
- Chickpea flour
- Almond meal
- Baking powder
- Baking soda
- Cornstarch

Grains and Pasta
- Brown, red, and black rice
- Wild rice
- Farro
- Couscous
- Quinoa
- Oatmeal (rolled, quick, or steel-cut)
- Teff
- Barley
- Whole-grain pasta
- Bean pasta
- Tortilla wraps (these freeze well)

Beans and Legumes
- Red and green lentils
- Split peas
- Canned or dried beans (black, kidney, pinto, navy, cannellini, great northern, etc.)

Fruits and Vegetables
- Apples
- Oranges
- Lemons
- Bananas
- Grapes
- Dried fruit
- Sun-dried tomatoes
- Jams and preserves (no sugar added)
- Onions
- Potatoes
- Dark leafy greens
- Garlic
- Ginger
- Broccoli
- Avocados
- Frozen fruits and vegetables

Soy Products
- Tofu
- Tempeh
- Soy curls
- Textured vegetable protein
- Soy sauce
- Miso

Nuts and Seeds
- Almonds
- Walnuts
- Cashews
- Flax seeds
- Chia seeds
- Hemp seeds
- Pumpkin seeds
- Sunflower seeds

Spices
- A wide variety of spices are available. Basil, oregano, thyme, cumin, turmeric, ginger, and cinnamon are good to have on hand.
- Garlic powder
- Chili powder
- Onion powder

Other Goods
- Pasta Sauces (low sodium, low sugar)
- Canned tomatoes, tomato sauce, tomato paste
- Hummus
- Olives
- Pickles
- Artichoke hearts
- Lemon juice
- Apple sauce
- Plant-based milks
- Coconut milk, low-fat
- Nut butters
- Vegetable stock (low sodium)
- Vegan Worcestershire sauce
- Vegan mayo

- Salsa
- Sriracha
- Vegan butters
- Nutritional yeast
- Dried seaweed: nori, arame, wakame
- Seitan
- Tahini
- Mustard
- Liquid aminos (coconut aminos are lower in salt, but sweeter)
- Vinegars (apple cider, balsamic, white)
- Vegan sugar (Sugar in the Raw, Florida Crystals, beet sugar, turbinado sugar, date sugar)
- Vegan honey
- Maple syrup
- Date syrup
- Arrowroot powder
- Meat alternatives (on a limited basis): Gardein, Tofurky, Beyond Burger, Impossible Burger, etc.

Food Storage

Here are some tips to keep your food items as fresh as possible:

1. Before refrigerating vegetables, dry them off with a paper towel or leave their storage bags partially open so they can breathe. Special containers for produce are available, such as the **OXO GreenSaver Produce Keeper**.
2. Learn how long different types of produce will last in the refrigerator. Leafy greens, mushrooms, and sprouts are more perishable; place them in the front as a reminder to use them within a few days. In general, they are best kept in the lower part of the refrigerator, where the air is cooler. The top shelf is a good place for leftovers.
3. Broccoli, cauliflower, cabbage, carrots, and Brussels sprouts will last longer.

4. Place small items such as ginger and shallots in one of the small compartments in the refrigerator door so they will not be overlooked.
5. Herbs can be kept fresh by rinsing and patting them dry, wrapping in a moist paper towel, and storing in a sealed bag or container.
6. Some produce, uncut, does not need refrigeration. These include potatoes, onions, garlic, tomatoes, squashes, peppers, and many fruits, such as apples, oranges, lemons, limes, melons, bananas, berries, nectarines, and peaches. Note: Do not place potatoes near onions, as they give off a gas (ethylene) that will cause onions to sprout and spoil faster. Avocados, best bought when still hard, can be kept at room temperature to ripen. Once cut or ripe, they can be refrigerated. Berries can spoil quickly in the refrigerator, so they are best kept at room temperature and eaten (with rinsing right before) within a couple of days. One way to keep them lasting longer in the refrigerator is to soak them in a 3-to-1 mixture of water and white vinegar, followed by a thorough rinsing.
7. Bread to be eaten within a few days is best kept at room temperature, with the rest put in the freezer.
8. Flour can be stored in the freezer in an air-tight container.
9. Place frozen vegetables and fruits in specific areas/levels of the freezer for easy access.
10. Nuts and dried fruits do not need to be refrigerated.
11. Homemade nut butters, as they do not have preservatives, are best kept refrigerated.
12. Dried herbs and spices should be stored in a dark, cool, dry place such as a pantry or a cabinet.

Equipment

In addition to basic cooking equipment and utensils, these are some items that are especially useful for food preparation in a vegan kitchen:
- Food processor
- High-powered blender, such as Vitamix®
- Electric pressure cooker, such as Instant Pot®
- Electric spice grinder
- Garlic press

- Mandoline slicer (with glove!)
- Good grater, zester, or microplane
- Spiralizer

These are a few specialty items:
- Sprouting kit
- Plant-based nut milk maker
- Food dehydrator (especially for raw vegan foods)

Remember that going vegan does not mean you have to purchase a bunch of new stuff. This section offers *suggestions* to assist you in maximizing the potential of your new food habits. In any case, your kitchen contents will continually evolve as you explore plant-based cooking.

3.3 Food Processing: Myths and Truths

While a healthy diet prioritizes plant foods as close as possible to their natural state, food processing is a valuable tool that helps us eat a wider variety of safe and nutritious foods and beverages. Industry groups, underqualified professionals, and digital influencers have sown confusion around food processing and nutrition by spreading half-truths and even outright wrong information. This, of course, prevents consumers from making well-informed food choices. That is why we dedicated two sections of this book to clarify important topics on food processing and food label interpretation. Our purpose is to correct misleading information and empower readers on their journey to a healthier lifestyle.

In the following dozen pages, we will do our best to cover essential concepts of processed foods in a straightforward and science-based way.

Basic Concepts of Processed Food

All foods that are not in their natural state have been processed to some degree. Apart from fresh fruits and vegetables, most foods are transformed to some degree from field to fork. However, many consumers view the term "processed food" negatively, not understanding that food processing is a tool that can be used for different purposes. Processing methods are frequently employed to increase food safety, diversity, and nutrient bioavailability. For example, fermentation is a great way to convert raw materials into tasty and nutritious products (e.g., wheat into bread or soybeans into tempeh). Alternatively, processing may be used to transform low-value ingredients into appealing but nutritionally poor products (e.g., soda and candy). While all the products illustrated in Figure 6 undergo processing, they exhibit tremendously different nutritional value.

Long story short: *Purpose* is crucial in food processing. Like any other tool (think of a knife, for example), it can be used to do good or bad. This is a vital concept we should all be mindful of for a healthy diet.

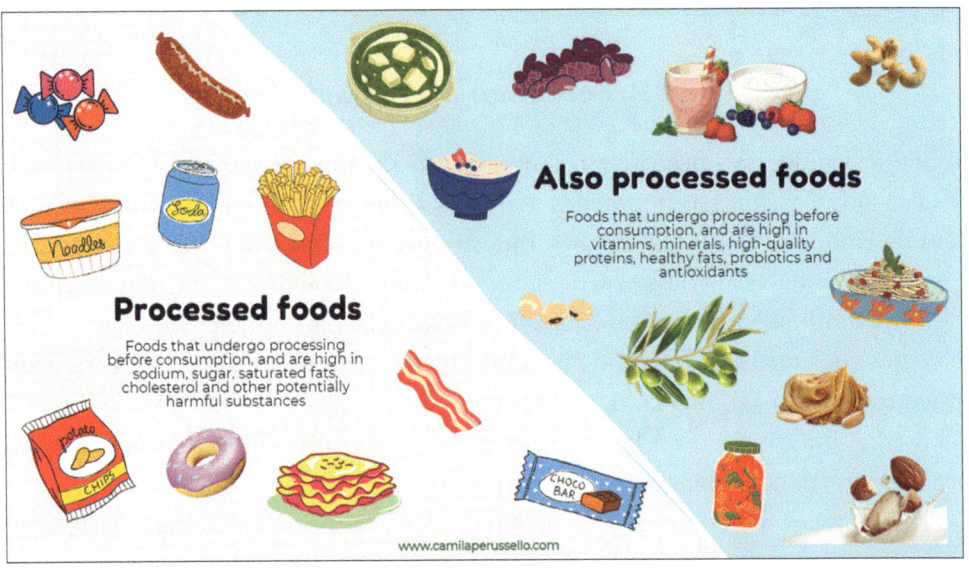

Figure 6. *Processed foods are not all the same. Source: www.camilaperussello.com.*

There are hundreds of processing methods as well as multiple ways food materials interact with processing factors to yield health benefits and risks. It is not by chance that food engineering is one of the most comprehensive fields in engineering.

We do not want to overwhelm the reader with complex information regarding the underlying mechanisms of food processing (this would be a topic for a whole new book—and a technical one). Therefore, we will clarify some central aspects of food processing by answering five common questions.

1. What is food processing?

Many people are surprised to hear that cooking is a form of processing—but it is. Many food technologies are processes that have been used for millennia to cook and preserve food, like salting, drying, and fermentation. Modern processing technologies involve both improved ancient methods and entirely new techniques, such as high-pressure processing and cold plasma.

In short, *food processing* refers to the set of methods and conditions applied to raw ingredients to transform them into consumable food products. It involves a series of mechanical, physical, or chemical processes that alter the form, structure, or composition of the ingredients, often to improve their safety, shelf life, taste, texture, color, or nutritional content. Food processing encompasses various stages, from cleaning and sorting raw materials to mixing, cooking, concentrating, separating, fermenting, enriching, preserving, packaging, and distributing the final products. This broad category of activities plays a crucial role in meeting the demands of a growing global population by providing a diverse range of nutritious, convenient, and safe food options, but it also raises concerns related to nutritional quality, additives, and potential health impacts. *Not all processed foods are the same*, and this must be clear to everyone.

2. Should we avoid processed foods?

Not necessarily. The nutritional value of a food item is influenced by processing—but sometimes for better, sometimes for worse. In addition, processing alone does not determine the health properties of a food or beverage.

Generally, minimally processed foods (such as fruits, vegetables, beans, nuts, and whole grains) tend to retain more of their micronutrients, fiber, and other beneficial compounds. That is why we highlight the importance of focusing on *whole* plant foods for optimal health. Meanwhile, highly processed foods often (not always) contain added sugars, salt, saturated fats, and additives. This results in lower nutritional value and, if consumed regularly, health concerns. However, this general idea is frequently misinterpreted; i.e., the more "natural" the better. This oversimplification would imply that untreated cashew nuts (which contain a potent toxin) are safer than treated cashew nuts or that raw meat is preferable to cooked meat.

Cashew nuts would not be edible without processing—steam roasting is required to inactivate a natural toxin called urushiol, which causes skin burns, rashes, and blisters. When we buy cashew nuts labeled as "raw cashews," it does not mean they are in their natural state. It just means the nuts have not been roasted a second time for flavoring purposes, and no salt or sugar has been added (only in this case are they labeled as "roasted cashews"). This is a clear example of how food processing helps us make the most of nutritious resources.

In other cases, processing can have a two-way effect, like in red meat. While cooking and smoking increase the edibility and safety of animal flesh, heat interacts with *naturally occurring* compounds in meat, forming carcinogenic compounds. For instance, heterocyclic amines (HCAs) are carcinogens that form when animal muscle is exposed to cooking temperatures (around 212°F–572°F). When curing salts are used (e.g., in bacon and ham), cancer risks further increase due to the interaction between these additives and the compounds *naturally* present in animal flesh. Such interaction gives rise to carcinogenic compounds like polycyclic aromatic hydrocarbons (PAHs) and N-Nitroso compounds (NOCs).

In further cases, processing is used to produce foods and ingredients that are nutritionally poor and do not even resemble the raw materials they are made of. For example, high-fructose corn syrup (HFCS) contains high amounts of free sugars, which can lead to health issues, including obesity, diabetes, and fatty liver disease. HFCS contains no essential nutrients and is usually a main ingredient in candy, cupcakes, cookies, and junk food in general.

Again, food processing is not inherently good or bad—it depends on its purpose. Another important aspect of the health impact of a food item is *what the food is made of*. The raw ingredients play a significant role in the product's health properties. Following a varied WFPB diet is the most efficient way of eating health-promoting foods and minimizing heavily processed items.

3. Is the processing degree important to the nutritional value of food? For example, ultra-processed foods are linked to health problems.

We already know that processed foods are not all the same, as multiple factors drive the nutritional value and safety of food. While processing methods and conditions can affect food's nutritional properties of food (for better or for worse), the processing level or degree is not an accurate determinant of its health impact. For instance, some ultra-processed foods (UPFs) can be healthier than minimally processed options, depending on their composition.

Here is a take-home message: The effect of processing methods on nutrient retention and the formation of both beneficial and detrimental compounds varies for different foods, processing conditions, and nutrients. In some cases, certain nutrients may become more bioavailable or easier to digest after processing—e.g., through the fermentation of soybeans into tempeh. In other cases, the interaction between food and processing factors (temperature, additives) can yield detrimental compounds—such as the formation of nitrosamines in cooked meat.

In summary, there is no direct relationship between processing degree and health outcomes. Let us elaborate on this by presenting four examples of food products with the *same intended use* but different processing degrees (Figure 7): legumes, steak, cured meat, and plant-based meat alternatives.

- **Legumes** (like beans, peas, and lentils) are considered **minimally processed**—they are usually dried or cooked and canned before consumption. These are wholesome foods that offer a range of health benefits.

- **Steaks** are "fresh" meat cuts derived from mammals, consisting of muscle fibers, connective tissue, fat, and blood vessels. Although they undergo several transformation stages from farm to table (e.g., killing, bleeding, evisceration, skinning, scalding, dehairing, deboning, cutting, chilling, etc.), they are classified as **minimally processed**. But unlike legumes (also categorized as minimally processed), steak consumption poses severe health risks, including cancer and cardiovascular diseases.

- **Cured meats** (like sausage, ham, and bacon) have curing salts added to prevent spoilage and to impart distinctive flavors and textures. They can also be smoked, which involves exposure to smoke from burning wood or other materials. This imparts a characteristic smoky flavor, enhances color, and contributes to the preservation process. Cured meats are classified as **moderately processed** foods. Not only are they proven carcinogens at the top class, Group 1 (WHO & IARC, 2015), but they are also rich in cholesterol and saturated fats.

- **Plant-based meat alternatives** (like bean burgers and soy sausages) are considered **ultra-processed**. Different plant-based meats exhibit different composition and nutritional value. In general, they offer good quality protein and dietary fibers with zero cholesterol and lower levels of saturated fat than their animal counterparts. Unlike real meat, plant-based alternatives are *not* associated with cancer risk.

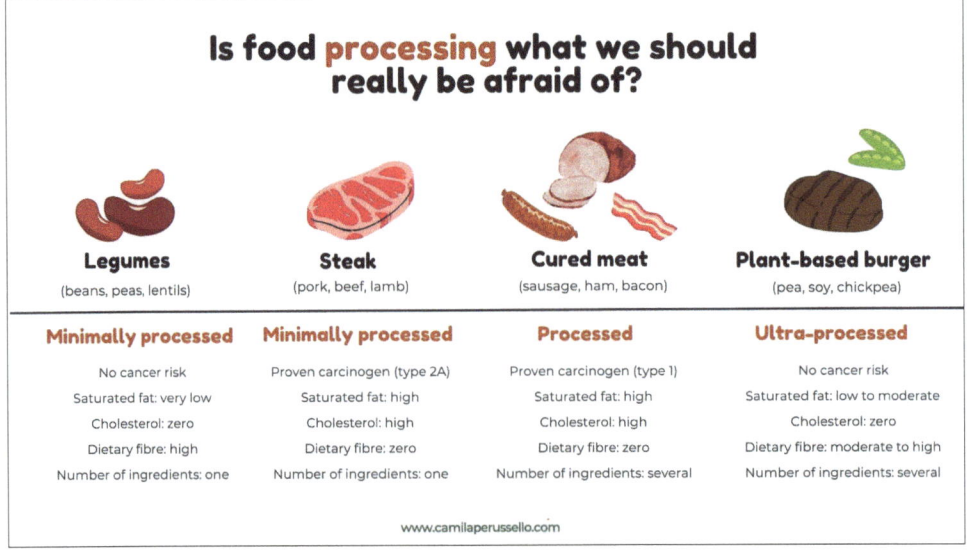

Figure 7. *Health impact of different foods: no direct relationship between processing degree and health outcomes. Cancer risk categories according to WHO & IARC (2015). Source: www.camilaperussello.com.*

These examples demonstrate that choosing one product over another based on their processing degree or number of ingredients is simplistic and inaccurate. But let us talk about UPFs specifically.

There is no legal definition or scientific consensus on what constitutes a UPF. However, many UPFs are made to be convenient and appealing to consumers while offering poor nutrition. UPFs are commonly rich in added sugars, saturated fats, refined starches, and sodium. Also, they typically contain additives to improve flavor, texture, appearance, and preservation. In the United States, nearly 60 percent of the calorie intake and 90 percent of the energy intake from added sugars come from UPFs that are calorie-dense and nutritionally poor (Steele et al., 2016). The overconsumption of UPFs is associated with a range of health issues, including cardiovascular problems, cancer, and metabolic diseases (Chen et al., 2020; Cordova et al., 2023). However, *not all UPFs are the same*. UPFs are a broad class that includes products with completely different compositions and nutritional values; for example, chicken nuggets and wholegrain breakfast cereals are both considered UPFs.

Painting UPFs (or processed foods in general) with the same brush regarding their health impact is tremendously imprecise and unscientific. While food processing and health are interconnected, condemning processed foods is a dangerous oversimplification that creates confusion among consumers.

In 2009, a classification system called **NOVA** categorized food items into four groups according to their processing level: 1) unprocessed or minimally processed foods; 2) processed culinary ingredients; 3) processed foods; and 4) ultra-processed foods (Monteiro, 2009). While NOVA does provide valuable guidance for healthier food choices, it fails to consider the basic principles of food processing engineering. For instance, it completely disregards the impact of different processing methods and conditions on specific raw materials and nutrients. The consequence? Consumers buy the misleading narrative of the meat and dairy industries that plant-based alternatives to animal products should be avoided because they are processed foods. In the meantime, cancer rates continue to soar (and animals continue to suffer).

From the perspective of food engineers—the most qualified experts in food processing engineering—the definition of UPFs by the NOVA system is inadequate, as there is no direct relationship between the number of ingredients or processing level and the nutritional value of food (Derbyshire, 2019; Knorr & Augustin, 2021; Petrus et al., 2021; Braesco et al., 2022). As discussed in a paper published in *Trends in Food Science & Technology*, "[k]nowledge of food engineering and/or science must be taken into consideration if food processing is the key for food classification. NOVA could be acceptable if it were based only on health concerns, but this was not the case" (Petrus et al., 2021). Luckily, science is constantly evolving and self-correcting, and many researchers have been proposing adjustments to the NOVA system.

Robust evidence shows that some UPFs can be healthier than less processed options (Cordova et al., 2023). That is because the composition of the raw ingredients in a food product largely determines its health impact. We have already mentioned a clear instance of two UPFs with entirely different nutritional values: wholemeal breakfast cereals and chicken nuggets. Now, let us see another example where two products with the *same intended use* are compared: animal flesh and plant-based meat.

While red meat products are proven carcinogens (**WHO & IARC, 2015**) and sources of saturated fat and cholesterol, plant-based alternatives have a high protein content, provide dietary fiber, contain much less saturated fat, are cholesterol-free, and pose no cancer risks. Nevertheless, according to NOVA, plant-based meat is considered a UPF. Again, a major result of the inconsistencies of NOVA and the misinformation on food processing is that the average consumer rejects healthier alternatives to conventional but harmful food products.

A recent multinational cohort study conducted with 520,000 participants in Europe investigated the health impact of UPF consumption. UPFs have been divided into nine groups, as seen in Figure 8. Significant differences in health impact were found between UPF groups, with the biggest risks associated with *animal products*. In contrast, ultra-processed plant-based alternatives, breads, and cereals were *not* associated with cancer and cardiometabolic diseases.

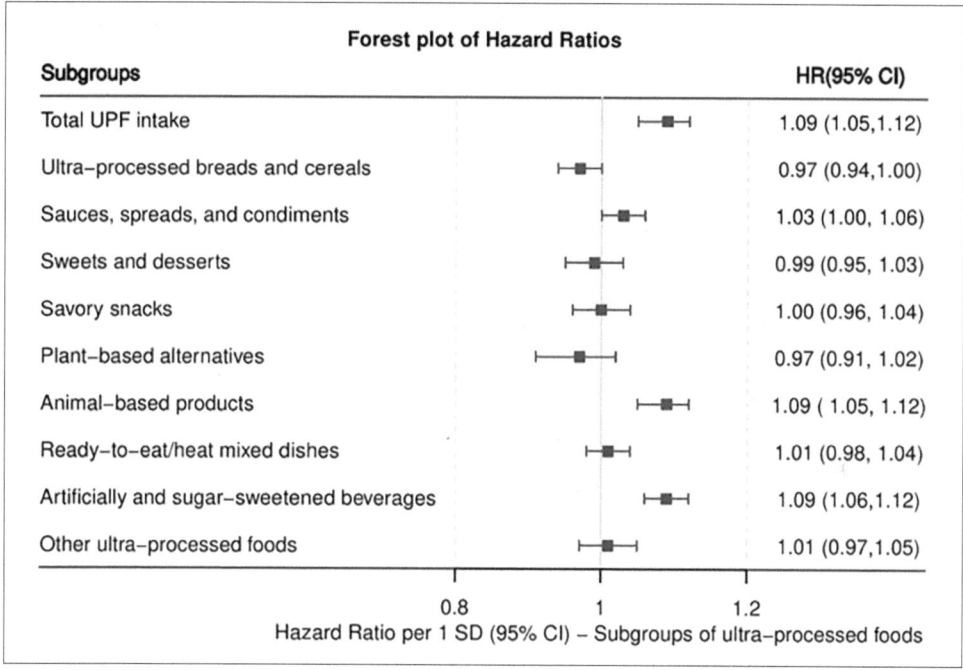

Figure 8. *Associations between subgroups of ultra-processed food consumption and risk of cancer-cardiometabolic multimorbidity. Source: Cordova et al. (2023). Abbreviations: HR, hazard ratio; CI, confidence interval; SD, standard deviation.*

Bottom line: no straightforward relationship exists between the food processing degree and health properties.

4. Do all processed foods contain additives?

Absolutely not. Additives are substances added to food for various purposes, such as improving taste, texture, appearance, shelf life, or nutritional content. Some common additives include preservatives, colorings, flavorings, stabilizers, and emulsifiers. Many processed foods contain additives, but many do not. As we have seen, the term *processed foods* encompasses a wide range of products, from minimally processed items like cut vegetables and roasted nuts to heavily processed and packaged convenience foods like chicken nuggets. The degree of processing and the presence of additives can vary significantly between different products.

Here is a general breakdown of processed foods based on their level of processing and additive content:

i. **Minimally processed foods**: These are foods that have undergone minimal processing to preserve their freshness and nutritional value without significantly altering their form or structure, like washing, cutting, and blanching. These often include whole foods like fresh produce, nuts, grains, and frozen fruits and vegetables. They typically do not contain added preservatives, colorings, or flavorings.

ii. **Moderately processed foods**: Foods in this category have undergone further processing but may still resemble their original form. They often involve more than one ingredient and may include cooking, fermentation, and other processing methods. Examples include canned beans, dried fruits, yogurt, many breads, and nut butters. While moderately processed foods may contain some additives for preservation or texture, the ingredient list is generally shorter.

iii. **Heavily processed foods**: These are convenience foods that have undergone extensive processing and may contain a higher number of additives. Examples include pre-packaged meals, snacks, and ready-to-eat items. Additives are often used to enhance flavor, extend shelf life, and maintain product consistency.

Many food companies opt for "clean label" ingredients, where synthetic additives are replaced with natural alternatives that provide similar effects on the product's sensory properties and shelf-life, such as apple cider vinegar, beetroot extract, and lemon juice. It is important for consumers to read food labels and interpret ingredient lists correctly, regardless of the presence of additives.

Some people choose to minimize their intake of heavily processed foods with a high content of additives, focusing on whole or minimally processed foods to support a more balanced and nutrient-rich diet. While we *fully* encourage this approach (and follow it ourselves), bear in mind that food additives are far from being the primary health concern in the average diet.

5. Should we avoid products with long ingredient lists?

Saying that products that contain many ingredients are unhealthy is as silly as saying that adding more fruit to your shake is bad. The number of ingredients says absolutely nothing about the nutritional value and health impact of a food or beverage. Again, the controversial NOVA system is primarily to blame for this misconception, as it groups foods according to the processing level and number of ingredients, conveying a false impression that fewer ingredients mean healthier food. Digital influencers with no knowledge of food technology and certain industry groups with vested interests reinforce the myths about food processing. Nutritional advice should be based on sound scientific evidence, and that is our purpose in this book. More details on food label interpretation are discussed in the next section.

3.4 Understanding Food Labels and Ingredients

Consumers usually get confused about the meaning of all the information printed on food packaging. Another concern is whether health and nutrition claims can really be trusted. This section will discuss food ingredients, additives, and health claims to help you interpret food labels and make better food choices. Once we understand some fundamental concepts, reading food labels becomes easy and even fun!

People commonly complain about all the work they must do to avoid unhealthy food. Quite frankly, that is because they focus on the *wrong* thing, on issues of secondary importance. For example, they look for a gluten-free microwave lasagna instead of naturally gluten-free foods, like potatoes, rice, quinoa, pulses, nuts, tofu, and veggies. By choosing the ready-to-eat meal, they will consume unnecessary calories, salt, fat, additives, and high glycemic ingredients. It is all the worse if the lasagna contains animal ingredients like eggs, milk, and meat. Another typical example is the concern with HFCS, a sweetener that replaces sucrose (table sugar). A high HFCS intake leads to tooth decay, increased liver fat, diabetes, and obesity.

However, note that HFCS is typically found in items like soda, sweetened dairy products, refined morning cereals, white bread, ice cream, cookies, frozen pizza, salad dressing, and so forth. Bottom line: If one is consuming too much HFCS, it is because they are consuming unhealthy food *in general*. Therefore, watch out for blaming a single ingredient when the problem is actually your diet as a whole.

Before we discuss food label information, let us understand some basic concepts about food packaging. Much research and technology goes into creating food packaging materials and designing packaging. Packaging helps contain the product, transport it over long distances, and keep it safe until consumption. Packaging also helps convey important information to the consumer, like expiration dates, nutrition facts, potential hazards (such as allergens), and the way the food was produced. Moreover, packaging increases convenience and serves a marketing purpose—beautiful packaging sells more! Beyond the visual appeal, strategic claims and wording can also convince people to buy one food item over another.

Basic Information on Food Labels

In the United States, the Food and Drug Administration (FDA) is responsible for food labeling. Basic information packaged foods must carry on the label includes the name and address of the manufacturer, packer, or distributor, the brand and name of the product, approved nutrient and health claims, the weight, volume, or count (depending on product type), the expiration date, and finally, the nutrition facts informing consumers of the number of calories and percentage of specific nutrients. In general, the more processed, the more information you will find on the label. This does not mean that produce cannot carry a label with meaningful information. By law, fresh fruits and vegetables do not need to have an expiration date; however, they can be labeled with health claims and other relevant information. Even the numbers on fruit and veggie stickers mean something important; for example, the growing method.

Meaning of Fruit and Veggie Stickers

You may have noticed that fruits and vegetables frequently carry stickers. What do the codes on these stickers mean, and why should we pay attention to them?

The numbers on the stickers are called Price Look-Up or PLU codes. There are approximately 1500 PLU numbers, each of which refers to a different type of fresh produce. The PLU numbers are standardized globally, meaning 4011 stands for conventionally grown yellow bananas anywhere in the world. These numbers help the cashier know what produce you are buying and the right amount to charge. The number does not necessarily indicate where the produce is from or who the producer is, but you often find this additional information on the label. Key information the consumer can obtain from the PLU number is whether the food is organic or conventionally grown, if it has been genetically modified, or if it's been treated with radiation to extend the shelf-life. For example:

- Fruits and veggies with four-digit numbers are conventionally grown (e.g., 4011 = conventionally grown yellow banana).
- Five-digit numbers starting with "9" are organic (e.g., 94011 = organically grown yellow banana).
- Five-digit numbers starting with "8" are genetically modified.
- Five-digit numbers starting with "3" mean that the produce has been irradiated to kill pathogens.
- Five-digit numbers starting with "6" are pre-cut produce.

Another important observation is that genetically modified produce does not need to be labeled as such, depending on the country. From the labels, the only way to be sure that the fruit or veggie is not genetically modified is by choosing organic products—organic production forbids genetically modified organisms (GMOs). More information about PLU codes can be found online on the PLU code database.

Some people are annoyed by seeing stickers on their produce, but we find them in most big supermarkets and grocery stores. You can avoid them by shopping at farmers' markets, organic food stores, community-supported agriculture programs, or, of course, growing your own food. On the other hand, the fact that the produce is labeled can be positive because you can track how it was produced. Buying food directly from the farmer is not necessarily safer, as you do not know how it was grown. Can we trust everyone?

Expiration Dates

Another important thing about food labels is the meaning of expiration dates. The two main expiration dates found on food labels are "best before" and "use by." These are associated with the reason why a food or beverage spoils. Different foods spoil for different reasons, for example, microbial growth, biochemical reactions, and physical reactions (like moisture uptake). Certain products might not have retained their best quality, like a stale cookie, but this does not mean that consuming it will cause harm. Other expired products might pose serious health hazards, like meat, dairy, and eggs carrying considerable counts of dangerous bacteria. That is why food legislation requires different expiration dates according to the product.

With those basic concepts in mind, "use by" dates refer to food *safety*. This means that one should not eat these products after the expiration date because microbial pathogens might be present in a dangerous number. In turn, "best before" dates refer to food *quality*, so one can still eat these products after that date. The difference is that the product might not be as fresh as before. Most animal products and other perishable foods carry a "use by" date, while plant-origin products like rice, dried pulses, canned fruits, frozen veggies, and chocolate carry a "best before" date.

Understanding date labels can help you avoid food poisoning, reduce food waste, and save money. Following the storage instructions is crucial to keeping food fresh and safe for consumption. If you leave a perishable product out of the fridge, for example, it will spoil before the date indicated on the label.

Important tip: If you go to the supermarket and see a discounted product near the expiration date, you can still consume it if it is stored properly. You must store it under proper storage and hygienic conditions and eat the food until its "use by" date—or even freeze it to extend its shelf-life beyond the expiration date. If a product is labeled with a "best before" date, the food might have lost its firmness, crispness, and consistency, but you may still eat it or repurpose it.

Other date labels sometimes appear on food packaging, such as "sell by" or "display until." These dates do not need special attention from consumers, as they are meant to help retailers control their stock. Moreover, labels like those are not even regulated. In conclusion, the most important labels to understand and look for are the "best before" and "use by" dates.

Health Claims

There are as many health claims as there are food products. Many are not mandated by legislation or even regulated—they are mostly used to attract consumers. Let us discuss the main health claims.

i. **Diet and light**. Consumers often get confused about the difference between those two labels. *Diet* products must have 100 percent of a specific ingredient removed or replaced with another ingredient. They are usually targeted at people with specific health conditions, like diabetes, high blood pressure, or high cholesterol. Diet soda, for instance, has no sucrose. In the meantime, *light* products have at least 25 percent of a certain ingredient removed or replaced with an alternative, or at least 25 percent fewer calories. Depending on the country, this percentage rises to 50 percent or more. Light products are usually targeted at people who want to reduce their intake of a certain ingredient or lose weight.

ii. **Sugar-free and zero sugar**. Products labeled as *sugar-free* or *zero sugar* will have the sucrose replaced with alternative sweeteners, which can be natural or artificial. Aspartame, stevia, sucralose, acesulfame potassium, xylitol, sorbitol, and mannitol are all examples of sweeteners. Some of these products can have zero or near zero calories, but attention—others may have *more* calories than the regular version. And that is because *sugar-free* products must contain less than 0.5 grams of sugar per serving but can still contain calories from other sources—other carbohydrates, fats, and proteins. Therefore, sugar-free (zero-sugar) products might not be suitable for diabetics and are *not necessarily* deprived of calories. On the other hand, the *zero-calorie* claim means the sweetener that replaced sucrose has nearly zero calories per serving.

iii. **GMO-free**. A product labeled *GMO-free* means the food and its ingredients have not had their DNA altered to meet specific characteristics, such as crops that are made resistant to insects. According to the WHO, GM foods are *not likely* to present risks to human health. The safety of GM foods is still up for debate within the scientific community because there are not enough long-term studies to draw definite conclusions. The only way to avoid GM foods is to buy 100 percent organic—which is unfortunately unrealistic for the vast majority of us. A crucial thing to remember is that GMO-free products can be either organic or conventionally grown, but all organic foods are GMO-free.

iv. **Free of artificial colors and flavors**. Foods and beverages that are free of artificial colors or flavors can still have added colors and flavors that were synthesized in a lab but are identical to the molecules found in nature. There are three main classes of additives: natural, nature-identical, and artificial. Regardless of the origin, all additives must undergo safety tests and be approved by national or regional legislation before use.

v. **Gluten-free**. As explained in a previous item, gluten-free foods are free from a protein called gluten, which causes allergies or sensitivity in certain people. Grains that contain gluten include wheat, rye, barley, spelt, and triticale (a cross between wheat and rye). A label that says "may contain gluten" means the food was processed in equipment that also processes foods containing gluten. In this case, there might be the risk of cross-contamination, but the percentage of gluten is often negligible and innocuous to most people. For safety reasons, manufacturers must warn consumers about this. If you have celiac disease, please *do not* consume foods with a "may contain gluten" warning, even if you do not see any gluten-containing ingredient on the ingredients list.

vi. **Whole-grain or whole-meal**. In their natural state, grains have different portions or "layers": the bran, the germ, and the endosperm. The bran contains much of the fiber, vitamins, and minerals of a grain. When grains are refined, the bran and germ (which are nutrient-rich but make up a small part of the grain) are removed, leaving the endosperm (which is basically made of carbohydrates). Therefore, whole grains are more nutritious than refined grains. When a product is genuinely "whole-grain" or "whole-meal," it retains more of the original fiber, vitamins, and minerals compared to its more refined counterparts. In so-called "enriched" products, some of the lost nutrients may be added back in, but not the fiber. Dr. Michael Greger describes his "5-to-1 Fiber Rule" as an easy way to determine if a product is whole-grain or not. From the information on the package label, divide the number of grams of carbohydrates by the number of grams of fiber. If the result is less than 5, then the product is whole-grain (Greger, 2015). By the way, sprouted breads are always whole-grain, but multi-grain products usually are not.

vii.   100 percent natural, all-natural ingredients, and variations. These claims are not regulated by legislation and definitely leave room for interpretation. In plant-origin foods, they usually refer to the absence of synthetic additives. Please be mindful that terms like *100 percent natural, free of artificial colors*, and *fat-reduced* are often slapped on foods that are not even healthy.

viii.   Organic and 100 percent organic. Products labeled *100 percent organic* are those made entirely from organic ingredients. In plant-origin foods, this means that the crops they are made of are free of pesticides, herbicides, and synthetic fertilizers. However, if the label says just *organic* as opposed to *100 percent organic*, it means that at least 95 percent of the ingredients are organic. In addition, a label that says *made with organic ingredients* must have a minimum of 70 percent organic ingredients. Keep in mind that *organic* is not synonymous with *healthy*. Organic foods can still be packed with fat, calories, sugar, and other harmful substances.

Food Additives

Food additives are substances added to foods and beverages to maintain or improve their freshness, safety, taste, texture, or appearance. Additives are used intentionally to perform a particular job—which consumers often take for granted. For example, additives can avoid the separation of fats in mayonnaise or improve the consistency of barista oat milk so it becomes thicker and foamier. Food additives have been used for centuries for preservation—for example, salt in meat and fish, sugar in jam, or sulphur dioxide in wine.

Consumers are frequently (and rightfully) concerned about their intake of additives and highly processed foods. Nevertheless, it is crucial to understand that not all processed foods contain additives.

Additives are sometimes needed to ensure processed food remains safe and in good condition from the farm or factory; during transportation to warehouses, stores, and supermarkets; and finally to restaurants and households. But at the mention of "food additive," many people imagine lab-made chemical substances with long names that are harmful to human health. The truth is that everyday ingredients like table salt, sugar, herbs, spices, and plant extracts can also be used as food additives.

Salt and sugar are actually two of the most widely used food additives. Salt, for example, has been used for centuries for food preservation. Obviously, the regular consumption of salt and sugar should be avoided. Herbs and spices are also common additives. For example, turmeric, paprika, black pepper, and rosemary leaves are used to make food more appealing and extend its shelf life due to their antioxidant and antimicrobial power while imparting health benefits. Other ingredients from plants are also additives, like beetroot powder to improve color and garlic extract to impart antioxidant properties. Also, many isolated chemical compounds found in nature, such as citric acid and ascorbic acid (also known as vitamin C), are used as food additives. These two substances are naturally found in citrus fruits.

Of course, many additives are indeed chemical compounds synthesized in a lab. The word "chemical" frequently evokes negative associations, but it is worth remembering that all components of our food, all plants, our bodies, and the whole world around us are made of chemical compounds. Even water (or dihydrogen monoxide) is a chemical compound! Plus, the fact that something was made in a lab does not make it more or less safe than a naturally occurring substance. There is no straightforward relationship between the *source* and the *safety* of a substance.

Additives are classified into three main groups according to their *source*. **Natural additives** are extracted from plants, minerals, and (unfortunately) animals. For example, natural vanilla extract (or vanillin) is used to improve the flavor of foods and beverages. There are also **nature-identical additives**, which mimic natural compounds, meaning they are copies of substances that exist in nature. An example of a nature-identical additive is ethyl acetate, which is used to give a fruit flavor to different products. And finally, there are **artificial additives,** which do not occur in nature—like ethyl maltol, often used to enhance the taste and smell of ice cream. But here is an important thing to remember: No matter the origin, all additives must undergo safety tests to ensure they are safe for consumption.

In terms of their *function*, food additives are classified into different groups. The main classes include the following:

1. **Preservatives**, which help extend the shelf-life of food by inhibiting the growth of bacteria, yeasts, molds, and other microorganisms. Examples include sodium benzoate, potassium sorbate, and nitrites.

2. **Antioxidants**, which prevent or slow the oxidation of fats and oils, helping avoid rancidity, off flavors, and nutrient loss in food products. Common antioxidants include vitamin C (ascorbic acid), vitamin E (tocopherol), soy lecithin, butylated hydroxyanisole (BHA), and butylated hydroxytoluene (BHT). Natural oxidants like vitamin C and varied phytochemicals are extracted from plants. They also reduce body inflammation and prevent cellular aging.

3. **Colorings** are added to enhance or restore the color of food lost during processing and preparation. They can be natural, derived from plants or minerals, or synthetic. Examples include beet juice powder, caramel color, and Brilliant Blue No. 1.

4. **Flavorings** are added to improve or modify the taste and smell of food, and these make up the greatest number of additives used in food production. Flavor agents can be natural (like herbs and spices), nature-identical (like ethyl acetate), or synthetic, such as monosodium glutamate (MSG) and artificial flavors.

5. **Sweeteners** are used to impart sweetness. They can be natural, like sugar (sucrose), agave syrup, and honey, or artificial, such as aspartame, saccharin, and sucralose.

6. **Emulsifiers** help mix ingredients that would normally separate, like oil and water. They contribute to the stability and texture of products, such as salad dressings and mayonnaise. Examples include lecithin and mono- and diglycerides. Emulsifiers like polyglycerol polyricinoleate (PGPR) and lecithin can also help improve the texture and consistency of food ingredients, such as chocolate used in confectionery products.

7. **Stabilizers and thickeners** improve the texture, stability, and consistency of food products. Many of them are derived from seaweeds. Common stabilizers and thickeners include agar-agar, pectin, and carrageenan.

8. **Acidity regulators** control and adjust the pH of food products. Citric acid, apple cider vinegar, tartaric acid, and sodium bicarbonate are examples.

9. **Humectants** help retain moisture and prevent foods from drying out. Common humectants include glycerol, sorbitol, and propylene glycol.

10. **Anti-caking agents** prevent the formation of lumps and improve the flow of powdered or granulated products. Examples include silicon dioxide and calcium silicate.

11. **Gelling agents** are used to give a gel-like consistency to certain foods. Examples include fruit pectin and agar-agar, a seaweed-based product used as a substitute for gelatin, which is animal-derived.

12. **Fortifiers and supplements** are used to enrich a product with essential nutrients that were either lost during processing or are naturally present in low concentrations.

13. **Miscellaneous** are a mixed group that comprises all other additives; for example, enzymes. Enzymes are proteins that trigger or speed up biochemical reactions. They are used for different reasons, such as to improve the dough in bakery products. Frequently, enzymes do not end up in the final product.

Needless to say, the use of food additives is only justified when it does not mislead consumers and their application has a technological need. Also, food manufacturers are mandated by legislation to list ingredients and additives.

Before approval, food additives are tested and proven safe for that specific use *at determined amounts*. The safety assessment includes acute, short-term, and long-term tests. The health risk of food additives is evaluated by the WHO and the Food and Agriculture Organization of the United Nations (FAO). Those risk assessments are conducted by an independent, international expert scientific group—the Joint FAO/WHO Expert Committee on Food Additives (JECFA). This means that only food additives that undergo a safety assessment and are found safe within specified limits can be used. This applies whether food additives come from a natural source or are synthetic.

Food legislation varies from country to country, with some being more flexible than others. This is partly because national authorities approve the use of food additives based on either the JECFA assessment or an internal evaluation. Moreover, different countries and regions follow different methodologies and evaluation principles (e.g., *probability* in the United States versus *possibility* in the European Union). This explains why food additive legislation is generally more conservative in Europe, where additives widely used in the United States are banned. Sometimes the inverse can occur; for instance, a food color called Ponceau 4R is banned in the United States but approved in the European Union (EU).

Food legislation is constantly amended to follow new scientific findings. The JECFA committee gathers annually to assess new studies and review conclusions and deliberations (WHO, 2023). Some additives that had been deemed safe for consumption for a long time have been shown to exhibit potential health effects. For example, new investigations indicate that certain artificial colors (e.g., sunset yellow and tartrazine) may increase hyperactivity in children. Although more research is needed to establish a clear connection, in the United Kingdom, food and beverages containing these additives must carry a warning on the packaging, while manufacturers are advised to use alternative colors (NHS, 2023).

In the United States, additives are listed by their name, while in other countries, they can be associated with specific numbers or codes. In the EU, for example, approved food additives are given a unique number prefixed by the letter E (the famous E numbers). Only after the additives are shown to be safe are they given an E number. In the EU, colors are assigned an E number from 100 to 199, preservatives are coded as 200s, antioxidants as 300s, sweeteners as 900s, and so forth. E numbers help consumers understand the function of that specific additive.

Every year, scientists worldwide investigate the adverse health outcomes of traditional and new food additives to expand current evidence and increase food safety. Studies show that the excessive consumption of food additives can lead to a range of health issues (especially in more vulnerable age groups), including headaches, allergic reactions, abdominal discomfort, ulcerative colitis, and cancer (Cao et al., 2020; Zhou et al., 2023). Research groups have been particularly active in elucidating the impact of additives on gut microbiota and its health ramifications. Plant-based food additives have been studied as safer and more sustainable alternatives to current practices (Zang et al., 2023).

Here is a takeaway message: By following a WFPB diet, one automatically excludes or minimizes additives. Also essential to know is that the health impact of food is as much related to the natural components in the raw ingredients as to the processing stages and additives. Minimally processed, additive-free products rich in cholesterol, saturated fats, and other harmful compounds are not necessarily healthier than foods containing studied levels of additives for improved safety and quality.

To finish this section, let us emphasize that we are not *whatsoever* dismissing the health risks of food additives or encouraging the consumption of UPFs. On the contrary. Our approach is to eat healthily (and ethically) and inspire others to do the same based on robust scientific evidence.

Nutrition Facts

When reading food labels, several key nutrition facts can provide valuable information about the health properties of a product. Here are important nutrition facts to pay attention to on food labels:

1. **Serving size**: The serving size indicates the amount of food or drink typically consumed in one sitting. All other nutrition information on the label is based on this serving size, so it is crucial to compare it to the amount you *actually* eat.

2. **Calories**: The total calories per serving number tells you the energy content of the food. This information is important for managing overall calorie intake.

3. **Macronutrients**: Pay attention to the amounts of macronutrients per serving, as follows:
    - Total Fat: Consider the total amount but also the type of fat (saturated, unsaturated, trans). Saturated and trans fats should be minimized to avoid heart conditions. Unsaturated fats are a great ally in reducing LDL cholesterol levels and providing essential fatty acids for both mental and physical health, especially polyunsaturated fatty acids like omega-3. However, remember that too much fat (even if "good" fat) can make you gain weight and be detrimental to your health.

    - Cholesterol: Cholesterol is found *exclusively* in animal products. As dietary cholesterol increases serum cholesterol levels, the ideal cholesterol intake for optimal health is zero.

    - Sodium: Keep an eye on your daily sodium intake, which can affect blood pressure. The usual recommended limit for daily intake is 2300 mg.

    - Carbohydrates: Look at total carbohydrates and the breakdown into dietary fiber and sugars. Choose foods with higher dietary fiber and lower (or preferably zero) added sugars.

    - Protein: Protein is essential for various bodily functions and assists with satiety, helping you ingest fewer calories. However, favoring protein-rich products high in sodium, cholesterol, or saturated fats is not a smart choice.

- Vitamins and Minerals: Some labels list the percentages of daily recommended intake for vitamins and minerals. Focus on essential nutrients like calcium, B vitamins, and vitamin D, and ensure the product contributes positively to your overall nutrient intake.

4. **Ingredient List**: Prefer products with whole, recognizable ingredients. Products that contain palm oil, coconut oil, hydrogenated oils, and especially animal ingredients are generally higher in saturated fats.

5. **% Daily Value (%DV)**: The %DV indicates how much a serving of the food contributes to your daily recommended intake of various nutrients. It is based on a daily intake of 2,000 calories, so adjust accordingly if your calorie needs differ. Generally, 5% DV or less of a nutrient per serving can be considered low, and 20% considered high.

6. **Added Sugars**: Look for added sugars in the ingredient list and the amount of added sugars in grams. The American Heart Association recommends limiting added sugars for overall health.

7. **Allergen Information**: Check for allergen warnings if you have food allergies or sensitivities.

8. **Nutrition Claims**: As mentioned previously, be aware of nutrition claims such as "low-fat," "high in fiber," or "reduced sodium." These can be helpful but should not be the sole factor in your decision-making.

Remember that individual nutritional needs vary, and it is essential to consider your *overall* diet and health goals.

Final tips on food label interpretation

Interpreting food labels correctly is a valuable skill for making informed choices that align with your nutritional needs. Here are five final tips on what information to focus on and what to avoid when buying packaged food:

i. **The order of ingredients matters**. Ingredients are listed by weight in descending order, meaning the first ingredient is found in the greatest amount. If a food starts with sugar, run away! As a rule of thumb, avoid foods high in added sugars and sodium, and those that contain synthetic additives.

ii. **Manufacturers must list the additives—do not exceed the daily maximum intake**. The ingredient list must include the code or name of the additives. Sometimes, both are present. Additives are generally found in small amounts, only enough to perform a specific job. That is why additives are usually at the end of the list. Beware, though: The low concentration does not mean they cannot harm if one consumes too much of that product. That is why daily recommended intakes exist. Also, new scientific findings may reveal that previously approved additives do pose health risks. Think of how many things we thought were harmless in the past and now seem absurd to us. That is what science is here for, to help us make intelligent decisions based on objective determinations instead of guessing or speculation. To be on the safer side, avoid foods full of additives.

iii. **Do not rely solely on health claims—read the ingredients list**. Foods labeled as "free of artificial additives" can still contain synthetic additives. If the chemical substance can be found in nature but was synthesized in a lab (such as flavors and colors), the product can still claim they are free of artificial additives because they are nature-identical.

iv. **Both macro- and micro-nutrients are important.** When buying packaged food or comparing two products, pay attention to the quantities of protein, total fats, carbohydrates, and dietary fiber. Consider also the *types* of fats and carbohydrates. Some products have equivalent total fat content, but entirely different fatty acid profiles. Look for products rich in poly- and mono-unsaturated fats and avoid those high in saturated fats, trans fats, and cholesterol.

v. **Do not obsess over protein intake.** Our society is obsessed with protein, as evidenced by the plethora of protein supplements and powders on the market. Choosing between two products based exclusively (or mainly) on their protein content is not a good way to ensure you are picking the healthiest alternative. Excessive protein is either used for energy, converted to glucose, or (if truly excessive) can contribute to fat storage when calorie intake exceeds energy needs. Be sure to eat plenty of whole foods rich in protein (like beans, lentils, tofu, and tempeh), and you will be fine.

In conclusion, our best advice to avoid additives and highly processed foods is to fill up your meals with fruits, vegetables, whole grains, beans, lentils, chickpeas, and other whole plant foods. This way you will get all the nutrients you need for optimal health with zero cholesterol and low levels of saturated fats and other potentially harmful substances. As a bonus, you will also lower your carbon footprint and the demand for products that harm our fellow animals. We can literally change the world when we know better.

3.5 Eating Plant-based on a Budget

In exploring diets and new ways of eating, it is natural to be concerned with food costs and what might be involved with food preparation. We constantly hear of the latest diet, quick weight-loss solution, superfoods, supplements, or ingredients that have seemingly made their way into almost everything. Think turmeric, for example—there are now turmeric cookies, crackers, lattes, and even oatmeal!

Food businesses reach out to potential consumers with the ultimate goal of making a profit, drawing on effective marketing strategies to create interest in new and improved products.

There is no doubt that the plant-based food market has seen phenomenal growth, even over just the past few years. The availability of plant-based products is no longer limited to only health food stores and specialty-item grocery stores; they are now found throughout regular supermarket chains and even convenience stores such as 7-Eleven. Food retailers are finding that the sale of plant-based products is bolstered when they are placed next to their conventional, animal-based counterparts. The plant-based label has even extended beyond food products. One sees a variety of household products proudly advertising they are plant-based—soaps, cosmetics, cleansers, and so on.

One of the many advantages of eating plant-based is a significantly lower grocery bill. Oftentimes we associate "special" diets with expensive ingredients and meal plans, but going plant-based leads to the pleasant discovery that not only is it healthier than a meat-centric diet, but it is also more affordable. You will notice your overall food costs decreasing as you reduce and eliminate animal products from your meals.

A few broad guidelines can help you get started. In creating grocery-shopping lists, it is strategic to prioritize the selection of whole plant foods and minimize the purchase of processed and packaged foods that are usually lower in nutritive value and more expensive. In doing so, one develops a keen shopper's sense of the best places to shop in terms of both quality and price. The shift from old, established shopping habits can become an exciting reacquaintance with food as one discovers and takes advantage of the extraordinary diversity of vegetables, fruits, whole grains, nuts, and seeds that are central to a vegan diet. The aim should be to, as they say, "eat the rainbow." All the beautiful colors of vegetables and fruits reflect the tremendous variety of phytonutrients that contribute to enhanced health and well-being.

Here are a couple dozen tips for eating plant-based on a budget:

1. By planning every week's meals with a shopping list, it will likely be easier to stay within budget.
2. Plan your meals so that ingredients can be used in multiple ways throughout the week.
3. A common piece of advice to avoid unnecessary spending is not to go grocery shopping when you are hungry!
4. Mainstream grocery stores often have their *own* lower-priced brands of stock items.
5. Be aware of when particular produce items are in season, with lower prices.
6. Explore local Asian markets, which often carry a wide range of inexpensive produce and harder-to-find varieties of vegetables and fruits that one might not find at a regular grocery store.
7. Packets of dried mixes for items such as falafel and veggie burgers are often cheaper than the ready-made versions.
8. See if your local grocery store has a section of marked-down, slightly blemished produce. These can be ideal for making smoothies.
9. Some stores will reduce prices as they near closing time.
10. Shopping in bulk can result in huge savings. Nuts, for example, can be up to three times the cost when purchased in a grocery store, compared to buying bulk online. Other bulk foods can include pasta, beans, rice, and seeds. Ethnic grocery stores often have spices in bulk.
11. As beans and lentils should be an important part of your vegan diet, it is a lot less expensive to purchase them dried.
12. Learn how easy it is to make WFPB foods that are healthier and considerably cheaper than stored-bought versions. These include hummus, nut butters, sauces, dressings, and even chips, salsa, and pesto.
13. Take advantage of companies that fight food waste by delivering "flawed" or surplus organic items and other food products at tremendous savings. Two such companies are Misfits Market (www.misfitsmarket.com) and Imperfect Foods (www.imperfectfoods.com). There are also companies such as Thrive Market (www.thrivemarket.com) that offer discount foods, as they buy at wholesale prices.

14. As you start making the transition to plant-based eating, "veganizing" some of your favorite dishes can result in savings right away as you switch out meat products with plant substitutes.
15. You can prepare meals that are not only inexpensive, but also delicious, simple, and quick to prepare. One dinner meal, for example, can consist of a simple homemade chili, whole-grain bread, and a salad of assorted greens and veggies, topped with drizzled vinegar and lemon juice.
16. Only do occasional purchases of processed plant-based meat and cheese substitutes; the costs of these and other convenience foods can add up, and they are not necessarily the healthiest.
17. Frozen vegetables and fruits are substantially less expensive than fresh ones, with virtually no loss of nutritional value.
18. Cook up large quantities of items (even doubling or tripling a recipe) with serving-size portions frozen in containers for future use. Some examples include pasta sauces, casseroles, soups, and stews.
19. Save leftovers from dinner and use them for lunch the following day, instead of making a new lunch meal.
20. While farmers' markets have become more and more popular, note that prices may not necessarily be less expensive than store-bought items. However, it is possible to negotiate on prices, and farmers will often drop their prices substantially near the end of the day.
21. Depending on your geography and climate, try growing your own food. There is something particularly fulfilling about planting and raising your own fruits and vegetables, and it can be as easy and small-scale as container gardening. One can also rent a small plot at a local community garden. Some vegetables, such as kale, can even be grown indoors with full-spectrum lights.
22. It is helpful to keep a notebook of easy recipes that are tasty, nutritious, and inexpensive. Also, keep a small notepad with you when shopping to keep track of prices at the various stores you visit.
23. While you will reduce your exposure to pesticides and antibiotics by eating organic, which is more expensive, it is also helpful to know the types of produce

that are safe to eat non-organic. Every year, the Environmental Working Group (EWG) publishes a Dirty Dozen™ and Clean Fifteen™ list: www.ewg.org/foodnews/about.php.
24. Eat out less. Obviously, it is cheaper to cook at home, with the added advantage that you know exactly what ingredients are going into your meal.

In the last two chapters, our focus has been primarily on food and nutrition. The upcoming chapter will delve into other essential aspects of a vegan lifestyle.

Chapter 4

Veganism Beyond Food

The word *vegan* was first coined by Donald Watson in 1944, with the following definition formally adopted in 1988 by The Vegan Society:

> Veganism is a philosophy and way of living which seeks to exclude—as far as is possible and practicable—all forms of exploitation of, and cruelty to, animals for food, clothing or any other purpose; and by extension, promotes the development and use of animal-free alternatives for the benefit of animals, humans and the environment. In dietary terms it denotes the practice of dispensing with all products derived wholly or partly from animals. (The Vegan Society)

Veganism, in its broadest meaning, embraces the tenets of *ahimsa*, the Buddhist and Hindu doctrine of recognizing the connections between all beings and refraining from harming others. It applies not only to actions and behaviors, but also to the cultivation of mindfulness and thoughts based on harmonious and peaceful intention. Therefore, vegans adopt additional practices beyond food choices to abstain from animal exploitation to the greatest extent possible.

As noted previously, it is impossible to know *every* single instance of animal use, as the exploitation of other animals is still pervasive. The commodification of animals is based on the idea that they are only units of production, and the accompanying for-profit mindset means that every part possible of an animal's body is used. With cows, for example, up to 40 percent of their weight makes up offal (non-meat parts of the body)—certain organs such as brains, liver, and tongues are used as food, while blood, bones, fat, feet, hair, and skin wind up in a wide variety of household goods, clothing, cosmetics, and other products too numerous to mention. These body parts are not mere byproducts; they can account for an astounding one-third of slaughterhouse profits (Pachirat, 2011). Extensive research efforts have been dedicated to finding profitable uses for all parts of animals. Alternatively, the wealth of the plant, algae, and fungi kingdoms warrants research on the use of all *their* parts, rendering animal-free foods and materials even more sustainable than they already are.

As you take the path of the plant-based lifestyle, you will become sensitized to how animal products have been adapted for use in an astonishingly wide range of items that we use every day. As with food ingredients and labeling, it is a gradual process of learning and discovering how you can make the most ethical choices as a consumer.

Let's look at some guidelines to assist you with the various components of vegan living.

4.1 Shopping Cruelty-free

In order to purchase items that have not been tested on animals, it is important to know that while in the European Union (EU) there are specific restrictions regarding the labeling of products as cruelty-free, in the United States, there are *no* legal definitions for either the "Cruelty-Free" or "Not Tested on Animals" labels. This can lead to vague or misleading information; for example, a product may not be tested on animals, but it is possible that some of its individual ingredients *are*. In addition, a specific brand that does not test on animals may be owned by a large parent company that *does* animal testing. Also, be aware that an item labeled "cruelty-free" is not necessarily vegan. For instance, some beauty products are not tested on animals (therefore labeled "cruelty-free") but contain animal-origin ingredients. Luckily, there are helpful websites with product guides that consumers can turn to, including www.ethicalelephant.com and PETA's Beauty Without Bunnies, at www.crueltyfree.peta.org.

4.2 Clothing, Accessories, and Shoes

Avoid clothes made from leather (including suede), silk, wool, cashmere, angora, fur, and jackets that use down as a filling. While satin is often made from silk, it can also be made from polyester or nylon. In addition to natural and synthetic materials, nowadays there are many varieties of "vegan leather" made from plant materials. Cork, pineapples, and even mushrooms (the root-like fibers called mycelium) are now being used in clothing as well as accessories such as purses, wallets, belts, and hats.

With footwear, there are many options available that do not use leather or suede; plant materials, canvas, and recycled plastic are more and more common. You will almost always see labels inside the shoes indicating whether they were made with leather or manufactured materials.

4.3 Cosmetics, Skincare, and Shampoos

Examining the contents of these products can be challenging as, more often than not, one encounters a long list of unfamiliar, scientific-sounding ingredient names. As with food items, many animal-free products are now providing a "vegan" label designation, but it is still helpful to familiarize yourself with some of the most common ingredients that are always or mostly animal-derived: hair, bristles, beeswax (cera alba), caprylic acid, carmine, casein, chitosan, cholecalciferol, collagen, elastin, estrogen (or estradiol), gelatin, glucosamine, guanine, honey, keratin, lanolin, oleic acid, panthenol, propolis, retinol, RNA, shellac, and squalene. In the case of ingredients that can be sourced either from plants or animals, sometimes the only way to know is to contact the manufacturer directly; these include biotin, glycerin, hyaluronic acid, lecithin, "natural sources," perfumes and fragrances, and stearic acid.

Fortunately for the consumer, a growing list of companies now offer cosmetics and beauty products that are both vegan and cruelty-free. Comprehensive guides can be found at www.shoplikeyougiveadamn.com and www.crueltyfree.peta.org.

4.4 Medicines and Supplements

While it has become easier and easier to be vegan where food and clothing choices are concerned, the field of medicine and supplements is particularly challenging. This is due to a lack of consistency with labeling and very little transparency regarding how ingredients are sourced and how extensively they are used. With supplements, the facts are startling:

50% of all supplement products contain at least one animal-derived ingredient. [. . .] We estimate that over 24 billion fish and 18 million cows, sheep and pigs are consumed each year to make supplement ingredients for the US market alone. If that's not shocking enough, these supplements are packaged in roughly 1.8 billion plastic pill bottles. Only about 30% of these bottles are recycled and 3% end up in the ocean. (Terraseed, 2022)

It is helpful to know the five most commonly found animal-sourced ingredients in supplements: magnesium stearate, gelatin, vitamin D (from sheep's wool), omega-3s (from fish oil), and bee pollen.

With medications, while most will have been tested on animals, we are starting to see some positive steps in the right direction. In the United States, the FDA Modernization Act 2.0 was signed into law in 2022. While not a total ban, it *does* remove the legal requirement that new drugs be subjected to animal testing prior to human trials. There are now organizations like VeganMed (www.veganmed.org) that certify animal-free products, providing an extensive list to help consumers.

The longstanding use of animals in medical research and testing is deeply flawed and problematic, raising ethical concerns over using animals for the benefit of humans. Over 100 million animals suffer agonizing deaths in laboratories every year. At the core of the issue is the degree to which animal studies are not reliably applicable to humans. "Research shows that 92% of drugs tested on animals are discarded during clinical research on humans" (Dimitras, 2021). Fortunately, alternative methods of testing are increasingly being developed, such as the use of human cell cultures (called "organs-on-chips"), human tissue samples, skin models, and computer simulations. While innovative technologies are certainly making a shift away from cruel research practices, there may be times when, for reasons of specific health considerations, we cannot avoid medicines or procedures connected to animal research. We need to remember as vegans that our intentions are to avoid the use of animals "as far as is possible and practicable." Note that this does not mean avoiding harm only when easy or convenient, but instead being aware that sometimes the possibility of making an ethical choice is not existent—for instance, you either die or use a life-saving drug tested on animals. Of course, situations like that are rare and do not make you less of a vegan.

4.5 Cleaning Materials and Detergents

The chemicals in cleaning products are often animal-derived, and particular ingredients can appear under different names. For example, oleyl alcohols (found in plants but also fishes) may be listed as Ocenol or Oleths. Products do not necessarily use the same ingredients from year to year, and in the United States, manufacturers are not required under federal law to fully disclose what is in their products. However, organizations like the Environmental Working Group (www.ewg.org) and Ethical Elephant (www.ethicalelephant.com) have made it much easier for consumers to find vegan, cruelty-free products. The latter group publishes online guides covering liquid dish soaps, liquid and powder laundry detergents, dishwasher detergent pods, and a wide range of household cleaning products.

4.6 Furnishings

While accurate vegan labeling is less established with furniture than with food products, the demand for animal-free, sustainable materials is definitely on the rise. Faux leather made from plant materials has become popular, as has vegan silk. Obvious materials to avoid are leather, silk, horsehair, sheepskin (for example, in rugs), wool, and down (in pillows). Vegan-friendly furniture companies have also created alternatives to animal-derived adhesives and glues.

4.7 Sports and Entertainment

As would be expected, vegans do not take part in hunting or fishing, and do not support zoos, aquatic parks, rodeos, horse races, and bullfights.

For a consumer new to veganism, navigating through all the product options can be overwhelming. It is not always possible to know if you are avoiding animal-derived ingredients 100 percent. In our everyday choices, we can remember that our goal is to practice compassion to the greatest extent that is practical and possible. Just by refusing to consume animals, each of us is already moving the needle toward a new model of lifestyle and choices grounded in empathy and justice. Start somewhere!

In the next chapter, you will find twenty-two questions we are commonly asked as vegans and animal rights activists. Hopefully, they will give you further clarity on the importance of veganism—and how easy and rewarding it is to lead a life of more compassion.

Chapter 5

Frequently Asked Questions

1. Where do I get my protein on a plant-based diet?

Getting enough protein on a plant-based diet is entirely possible by incorporating a variety of plant-origin protein sources into your meals. Note that all foods and beverages are composed of different percentages of water and three main macronutrients: proteins, fats, and carbohydrates. Here are some excellent sources of plant protein:

Legumes: Beans, lentils, chickpeas, peas, peanuts, and lupins are protein-rich. They can be used directly in soups, stews, burritos, and salads. Legumes can also be made into burgers, falafel, Bolognese sauce, omelettes, and pancakes or consumed as butter and spread (e.g., peanut butter). In the supermarket, you can also find legume-based pasta, which is protein-rich and often gluten-free. This is an additional way of incorporating high-quality protein into your meals. Legumes like peanuts and lupins are also great protein-rich snacks. Lupins contain around 40 percent protein! They are still unknown in some parts of the world but are highly consumed in Mediterranean and Latin American countries. In fact, lupins are one of the most popular snacks in Portugal, where they are salted and pickled (*tremoços*).

Tofu and tempeh: Tofu and tempeh are versatile protein sources made from soybeans. Tofu, for example, contains around 17g of protein in 100g, all essential amino acids in good proportions, and a wide range of other nutrients. You can marinate and cook tofu and tempeh in various ways to suit your taste. You can make them into steaks and "chicken" pieces or use them in tacos, burritos, curries, and sandwiches. Another way to use tofu is in quiches and omelettes.

Seitan: Seitan is a high-protein meat substitute made from wheat gluten. It has a chewy texture and can be used in dishes like stir-fries and sandwiches.

Whole grains: Quinoa, brown rice, wild black rice, oats, barley, and bulgur are not only good sources of complex carbohydrates but also contain protein. Swapping cooked white rice (mostly starch) with cooked quinoa is an excellent way to add nutrition to your meals per kilocalorie, including essential amino acids. Whole-wheat pasta and bread also contain significant amounts of protein.

Nuts and seeds: Almonds, chia seeds, pumpkin seeds, sunflower seeds, flaxseeds, and hemp seeds are packed with protein. They can be eaten as snacks, added to smoothies, or used as toppings in salads, oatmeal, and various dishes. Nut and seed butters like almond butter and tahini (made from sesame) are also good options. Besides protein, nuts, seeds, and derivatives offer significant amounts of fiber, vitamins, minerals, and polyunsaturated fats (including omega-3 and omega-6).

Plant-based milk: Soy milk is one of the plant-based milks with the highest protein content since soybeans are legumes (legumes are the top protein-rich foods in the plant kingdom). Other legume-based milks, like pea milk, are equally good protein sources, although they are less common in the market. Although other plant-based milk alternatives, like almond milk, oat milk, and rice milk, have a lower to negligible amount of protein, they can be rich in other essential nutrients or be fortified with protein and vitamins, making them a good addition to your diet.

Soy products: Besides tofu and tempeh, soy-based products like edamame, soy yogurt, and soy-based meats can be good protein sources.

Vegetables: While not as protein-dense as other plant-origin sources, vegetables like spinach, asparagus, Brussels sprouts, broccoli, and artichokes still contribute to your overall protein intake.

Fruits: Just like vegetables, fruits contain some protein, but the amount is usually smaller than other plant-based protein sources. Some fruit sources of protein include passion fruit, dried apricots, raisins, avocado, and jackfruit. These fruits provide 3g–5g of protein per cup.

Plant-based protein powders: You can also incorporate protein powders derived from sources like pea, soy, rice, or hemp into smoothies and shakes. These products are made from the protein portion of the plant, meaning that much of the fat and carbohydrates have been removed. Plant-based protein powders typically provide 20g–27g of protein in 30g, other than vitamins and minerals like iron and vitamin K. Some powders are also good sources of probiotics, prebiotics, omega-3, and omega-6, which are beneficial for brain health and gut health. However, do not overindulge, as protein powders make it very easy to exceed our daily recommended protein intake. Excessive protein consumption can lead to detrimental health effects, including kidney damage and digestive issues. Additionally, some protein powders may contain additives that could have adverse health upon exaggerated consumption. Instead, prioritize obtaining protein from whole plant foods whenever possible.

Nutritional yeast: Nutritional yeast is a deactivated strain of *Saccharomyces cerevisiae* (the same microorganism used to make beer and bread). It is found in the form of yellow flakes or powder. Not only is nutritional yeast an excellent protein source (up to 50g of protein in 100g), but it is also one of the few natural sources of vitamin B_{12} that is animal-free. Nutritional yeast can also be fortified with B_{12} for additional nutrition. It offers good amounts of B-complex vitamins (up to 1000 percent of B_{12}, B_6, B_2, and B_1 daily needed intake!), calcium, thiamin, iron, and potassium. Nutritional yeast can be added to a wide range of recipes (e.g., quiches, omelettes, creamy white sauce) or be used as a topping to add color and a cheesy, nutty flavor. Try it with pasta or popcorn!

Meat alternatives: Plant-based burgers, sausages, bacon, and ham are usually made from legumes and grains, most commonly including soy, peas, chickpeas, and wheat gluten (although many can be gluten-free). Meat alternatives have a good protein content and can be used in recipes the same way you would use animal meat. The composition and, therefore, the nutritional value of plant-based meat varies considerably among products—for example, lentil patties versus a hyper-realistic, high-tech burger substitute. However, peer-reviewed studies show that meat alternatives can be part of a healthy diet and offer health benefits compared to animal flesh (PAN, 2023).

Modern society is obsessed with protein intake, yet protein deficiency is extremely rare (unless you are severely malnourished). In the meantime, a significant portion of the global population is deficient in *fiber* and *essential nutrients* like omega fatty acids, vitamins, and minerals typically found in plant foods. According to the USDA Dietary Guidelines, approximately 90 percent of the US population does not meet the daily recommendation of vegetables! The USDA recommends that adults consume around 45g–60g of protein from different sources per day—the exact amount depending on sex, weight, age, activity level, and life circumstances (e.g., pregnancy and lactation). In North America, Europe, Argentina, and Brazil, the average person consumes nearly twice the protein needed, mostly animal-sourced (Ranganathan et al., 2016). Robust evidence confirms that dietary changes toward fewer animal products and more plant foods improve nutritional status and overall health (Springmann et al., 2021).

Furthermore, consuming too much protein can affect your health negatively, especially in the case of animal-sourced protein. Animal products tend to be high in cholesterol and saturated fat and very low in digestive fiber, which are top factors in the development of metabolic syndrome and heart disease. Excess protein intake is associated with renal function problems and cardiovascular events, especially in the case of high protein-low fiber diets (Xu et al., 2016).

Moreover, as important as the *amount* of protein we ingest is the *type* of protein. Proteins are formed by smaller blocks called amino acids, some of which are not produced by the human body—those are called *essential* amino acids. This means we need to get them from outside sources. There is a total of twenty amino acids, out of which nine are essential amino acids—histidine, isoleucine, leucine, lysine, methionine, phenylalanine, threonine, tryptophan, and valine. In addition, protein-rich foods do not contain all amino acids in equal proportions, regardless of their source (Figure 9).

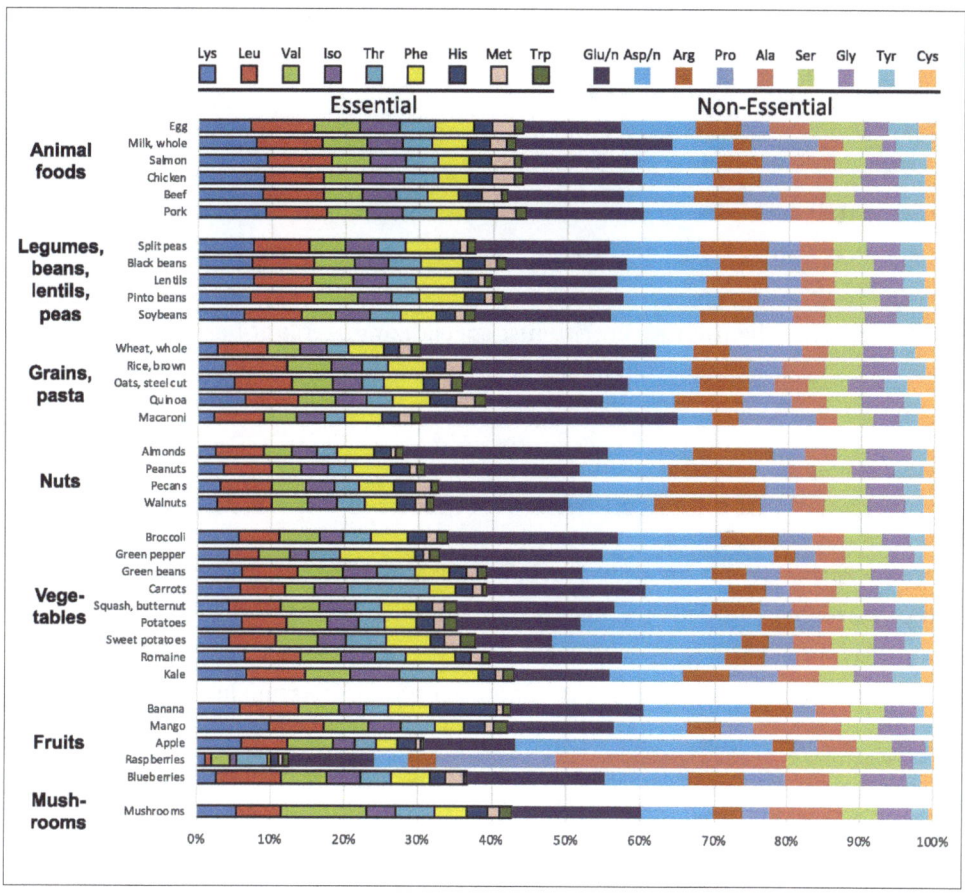

Figure 9. *Proportions of amino acids in selected foods across food groups. Source: Gardner et al. (2019). Abbreviations: Ala, alanine; Arg, arginine; Asp/n, aspartate and asparagine; Cys, cysteine; Glu/n, glutamate and glutamine; Gly, glycine; His, histidine; Iso, isoleucine; Leu, leucine; Lys, lysine; Met, methionine; Phe, phenylalanine; Pro, proline; Ser, serine; Thr, threonine; Trp, tryptophan; Tyr, tyrosine; Val, valine.*

Plants and algae produce amino acids through photosynthesis, which is the reason why humans do *not* need animal products for protein or essential amino acid intake (some of the largest animals are herbivores, right?). Animals only *metabolize* amino acids; they do not produce them.

The idea that only animal products provide "complete" proteins is incorrect, as plants, algae, and mushrooms do contain all essential amino acids, varying only in distribution or percentage (Gardner et al., 2019). By including different protein-rich plant foods in your diet, you can perfectly obtain all the protein and essential amino acids needed for good health.

By the way, the USDA recommends varying your protein source to ensure you ingest a wide range of other important nutrients, not only proteins. Incorporating a mix of the plant protein sources mentioned earlier will help you to meet your protein (and amino acids) needs and also to ingest minerals, vitamins, fiber, and essential fatty acids.

A registered dietitian or nutritionist specializing in plant-based nutrition can help plan a well-balanced plant-based diet that meets your protein and overall nutritional needs.

2. Will I get calcium deficient if I quit dairy?

Dairy products are not the only source of calcium; there are plenty of other foods that can provide you with the necessary calcium intake. Whether or not you will become calcium deficient after quitting dairy depends on your *overall* diet. Moreover, calcium deficiencies are frequently found across all diets, including vegan, vegetarian, and omnivore (Neufingerl & Eilander, 2022).

Getting enough calcium on a plant-based diet is absolutely possible by including a variety of calcium-rich plant foods in your meals. Here are some examples:

Leafy greens: Foods like spinach, collard greens, kale, broccoli, cabbage, Brussels sprouts, and bok choy (or pak choy) are excellent sources of calcium and many other vitamins and minerals.

Fortified plant-based milk: Many plant-based milk alternatives, like almond milk, soy milk, and oat milk, are fortified with calcium and other nutrients. Check the labels to ensure they contain a significant amount of calcium, but do not worry if they do not, as you can combine different sources of calcium in your diet. Again, the mineral does not have to come from a single food or beverage.

Nuts, seeds, and derivatives: Incorporate nuts and seeds into your meals and snacks. Almonds, chia seeds, and sesame seeds contain calcium as well as vitamins, minerals, fibers, and poly-unsaturated fats that contribute to overall health and good energy levels. Nut butters and seed spreads (e.g., tahini) are also great sources of calcium.

Tofu: Tofu is high in protein and contains all nine essential amino acids. It also provides unsaturated fats, high-quality carbohydrates, and a wide variety of important vitamins and minerals, like copper, calcium, and manganese. The exact nutrient content of tofu varies depending on the type of coagulant used to make it, as soymilk is coagulated to become tofu (similarly to cheesemaking). If you are concerned with your calcium intake, give preference to tofu that was set with calcium sulfate. Calcium sulfate–set tofu contains more calcium than nigari-set tofu, offering around 53 percent of the recommended daily value in 100g of tofu.

Legumes: Beans, lentils, and chickpeas provide calcium and other essential nutrients.

Whole grains: Foods like amaranth, quinoa, seeded bread, and fortified whole-grain bread can increase your calcium intake.

Dried fruits: Dried figs, apricots, and raisins are rich in calcium.

Fortified foods: Some foods, such as orange juice, plant-based yogurt, breakfast cereal, and nutritional yeast, are fortified with calcium. Check the labels for information on calcium content.

Seaweed: Some types of seaweed, like kelp, contain calcium. They can be consumed as a snack or as a spice in salads, soups, and other dishes. Sea vegetables are also an excellent source of dietary iodine.

Calcium supplements: You can also consider taking calcium supplements, but it is recommended to try to get nutrients from whole foods first.

If you are concerned about calcium bioavailability, it is worth mentioning that studies show similar calcium absorption between dairy products and plant foods like tofu, broccoli, and kale (Melse-Boonstra, 2020; Weaver et al., 2002; Heaney et al., 1993). Moreover, calcium-set tofu and Brassica vegetables (like Brussels sprouts) are *concentrated* sources of bioavailable calcium (Melse-Boonstra, 2020; Weaver et al., 2002).

It is also important to focus on nutrients that aid calcium absorption, such as vitamin D and magnesium. Spend some time in the sun (twenty minutes per day, if possible) or consider foods fortified with vitamin D.

As with any diet, balance and variety are key to ensuring you get all the nutrients you need. If you are struggling to get enough calcium from food sources alone, consider discussing calcium supplements with a healthcare professional.

3. Aren't vegans iron deficient?

Iron is an essential mineral that plays a crucial role in carrying oxygen throughout the body. Vegans can be at a higher risk of iron deficiency compared to individuals who consume animal products, but this does not mean vegans will become iron deficient. Moreover, iron deficiency can affect anyone, regardless of their diet (Neufingerl & Eilander, 2022). A balanced plant-based diet can provide all the necessary iron for optimal health.

It is important to mention that there are two forms of dietary iron: heme iron (found in animal products) and non-heme iron (found in plant-based foods). Non-heme iron from plant-based sources is not as easily absorbed by the body as heme iron from animal sources. Additionally, plant foods often contain compounds like phytates and polyphenols, which can inhibit iron absorption. However, excess heme iron can contribute to several health issues. It is linked to diseases such as hemochromatosis, cardiovascular disease, type 2 diabetes, liver cirrhosis, neurodegenerative conditions like Alzheimer's and Parkinson's, and certain cancers, especially colorectal cancer. Unfortunately, many people are unaware that high iron levels can promote oxidative stress and inflammation, damaging various organs and tissues. Therefore, consuming too much iron (especially heme iron from animal sources) is as problematic as consuming too little iron.

Many plant foods are rich in iron. Iron-rich plant foods include legumes (e.g., beans, lentils, chickpeas), tofu, tempeh, quinoa, fortified cereals, nuts, seeds, dark leafy greens (e.g., spinach, kale), and dried fruits. Make sure you include these in your diet. In addition, some strategies can be used to maximize iron absorption:

Combine iron with vitamin C: Vitamin C enhances the absorption of non-heme iron. Pair iron-rich foods with sources of vitamin C, like citrus fruits, bell peppers, strawberries, and broccoli. For example, eat an orange after a bean chilli or add broccoli and sesame seeds to a tempeh stir-fry.

Avoid inhibitors: Some compounds can inhibit iron absorption. Avoid consuming tea and coffee along with meals containing iron-rich foods, as those can hinder iron absorption.

Cooking methods: Certain cooking methods can enhance iron absorption. For example, soaking and sprouting legumes, as well as cooking them in a slightly acidic medium (e.g., containing vinegar or lime), can improve iron bioavailability.

Iron-fortified foods: Consume foods that are fortified with iron, such as fortified cereals, plant-based milk, and nutritional yeast.

If you are at risk of iron deficiency or have difficulty meeting your iron needs through diet alone, consider discussing iron supplements with a healthcare professional. Regular check-ups are also important, regardless of one's dietary habits, to detect potential deficiencies early.

4. Vegans must supplement with B_{12}. Doesn't this mean a plant-based diet is unhealthy?

The recommendation for vitamin B_{12} supplementation in a plant-based diet is not an indicator of an unhealthy diet, but rather a recognition that vitamin B_{12} is predominantly found in animal products. This vitamin is produced by *microorganisms* (*not* animals), which are present primarily in the soil but also in the intestines of human and non-human animals, especially ruminants (e.g., cows and sheep). Please note that most animals exploited for food (birds, pigs, and fishes) are *not* ruminants. Also, while food and water sanitation is obviously crucial to food safety, it lowers our gut counts of B_{12}-producing microorganisms to negligible levels (Perussello, 2022). Therefore, humans must get B_{12} from dietary sources and/or supplementation for adequate blood levels.

It is worth noting that we have been supplemented with vitamins and minerals our whole lives without realizing it. For example, the fortification of wheat flour with iron, zinc, and folic acid is recommended or even mandated by legislation in many countries, such as Brazil and the United Kingdom. In fact, the fortification of wheat flour with vitamins and minerals is a public health strategy promoted by the WHO (WHO, 2019). As for B_{12}, non-vegans are also supplemented indirectly, as farmed animals receive B_{12} supplementation regularly to meet production targets.

Vitamin B_{12} is essential for brain health, nerve function, and the formation of red blood cells. While it is true that vegans need to be mindful of their B_{12} intake, it does not imply that a plant-based diet is inherently inadequate, especially considering the *enormous* health benefits attributed to the WFPB diet over other diets (Springmann et al., 2018b; Wang et al., 2023).

It is important to understand that B_{12} deficiency is not unique to vegans; it also affects individuals who consume animal products. In addition, many omnivores may have adequate B_{12} levels due to animal products product, *as well as* fortified foods or supplements. To sum up, B_{12} deficiency is a concern for people *regardless* of their dietary preferences.

A balanced plant-based diet can be rich in essential nutrients, fiber, antioxidants, and phytochemicals that contribute to overall health and longevity. In fact, a robust body of evidence demonstrates that varied plant-based diets focused on whole foods are the most effective way of lowering the risk of cardiovascular disease, diabetes, high blood pressure, stroke, cancer, metabolic syndrome, and cognitive decline (Perussello, 2022).

Like any diet, nutritional balance and *variety* are key to a healthy plant-based diet. This involves incorporating a wide range of plant-based foods that provide various nutrients. Many plant-based foods are fortified with B_{12}, such as plant-based milk, cereals, and nutritional yeast. Supplementation is also a reliable and convenient way to meet this nutritional need without relying on animal sources or worrying about the overall content of B_{12} in your diet due to the fortified products you consume.

A vegan diet can provide numerous health benefits while ensuring adequate nutrition. It is important for anyone, vegan or not, to consult with medical professionals or registered dietitians to ensure they are meeting their nutritional needs. Please note that most healthcare professionals are still learning about the benefits of plant-based nutrition over traditional ways of eating, so make sure to find someone specializing in plant-based diets.

5. What plant-based foods are rich in omega-3 and omega-6?

Both omega-3 and omega-6 are essential polyunsaturated fatty acids (PUFAs) that our bodies need for various functions. The daily intake and also the ratio between omega-3s and omega-6s matter. A good ratio (ideally 1:1) improves brain health and exerts protective cardiovascular effects. The following is a list of plant-based foods that are rich in omega-3 and omega-6:

Foods Rich in Omega-3 Fatty Acids:

- **Flaxseeds** are one of the best plant-based sources of alpha-linolenic acid (ALA), an omega-3 fatty acid. One teaspoon of flaxseeds (approximately 28g) offers 6,388mg of ALA. Flaxseeds can be added to salads, breads, smoothies, yogurt, oatmeal, and overnight oats.

- **Hemp seeds** provide a good balance of omega-3 and omega-6 fatty acids and can be sprinkled on salads and yogurt, or blended into smoothies. They offer 6,000mg of ALA in 28g.

- **Chia seeds** are another great source of ALA omega-3 fatty acids, and they can be used just like flaxseeds. A portion of 28g of chia seeds offers 4,915mg of ALA.

- **Walnuts** contain a decent amount of ALA omega-3s and can be included in your diet as a snack or be added to various dishes. Walnuts offer 2,542mg of ALA in 28g (approximately five halves).

- **Brussels sprouts** (cooked) contain around 270mg of ALA per cup.

- **Algal oil supplements** are an excellent source of both eicosapentaenoic acid (EPA) and docosahexaenoic acid (DHA), which are the primary forms of omega-3 fatty acids found in fish. They offer 200mg–600mg of EPA and DHA in one to two soft gels. Fishes are rich in omega-3s because they feed on algae.

- **Seaweed** of certain types, like nori, is a source of omega-3s. They can be used in sushi rolls or be added to soups.

- **Soybeans** and soy products like tofu and tempeh contain small amounts of ALA omega-3s.

Foods Rich in Omega-6 Fatty Acids:

- **Sunflower seeds** are high in linoleic acid, a type of omega-6 fatty acid. They can be used in salads, breads, oatmeal, smoothies, and as a topping on dishes in general.

- **Safflower oil** is rich in linoleic acid and can be used for cooking or in salad dressings.
- **Sesame seeds** and derivatives, like sesame oil and tahini, are additional sources of omega-6 fatty acids. Sesame oil is often used for flavor in Asian cuisine.

- **Pumpkin seeds** contain linoleic acid and can be enjoyed as a snack or be added to salads, oatmeal, breads, and varied dishes.

- **Walnuts** provide omega-3 and some omega-6 fatty acids.

- **Pine nuts** are a source of omega-6 fatty acids that can be used in various recipes, including basil pesto.

- **Soybean oil** is commonly used for cooking and contains omega-6 fatty acids.

You might have noticed that we did not detail the content of omega-6 fatty acids in the listed foods as we did with omega-3s. That is because modern diets provide a much higher intake of omega-6s relative to omega-3s (Perussello, 2022; Micha et al., 2014). Although the ideal ratio between omega-6 and omega-3 is 1:1, the average ratio in the Western world is 16:1! This imbalance can be inflammatory to your body and detrimental to your overall health. Do not obsess with the ratio, however. You can maintain a healthy balance by incorporating sources of omega-3s into your diet and focusing on varied whole-plant foods.

If you are considering adding supplements to your diet, it is a good idea to consult with a healthcare professional specializing in plant-based diets to ensure you are making choices appropriate for your individual needs. However, dietary sources of omega-3 fatty acids are preferable to supplements, as the scientific evidence on their benefits is not conclusive.

6. Is it safe to eat plant-based during pregnancy and lactation?

Yes, it is safe to follow a plant-based diet during pregnancy and breastfeeding. As with any other diet, careful planning is required to ensure that both the mother and the baby receive adequate nutrients. According to the US Academy of Nutrition and Dietetics, "appropriately planned vegan diets are healthful, nutritionally adequate, and may provide health benefits for the prevention and treatment of certain diseases. These diets are appropriate for all stages of the life cycle, including pregnancy, lactation, infancy, childhood, adolescence, older adulthood, and for athletes" (Melina et al., 2016).

Here are some key considerations for a balanced vegan diet for pregnant and breastfeeding women:

Calories: Ensure you are consuming enough calories to support both your nutritional needs and the increased energy demands during pregnancy and lactation.

Hydration: Staying hydrated is essential for pregnant and breastfeeding women. Water, herbal teas, and fruit juices can contribute to your daily fluid intake.

Protein: Plant-based protein sources, such as beans, lentils, tofu, tempeh, nuts, seeds, and whole grains, can provide adequate protein during pregnancy and lactation. Ensure that you consume a variety of these protein sources to get a wide range of amino acids.

Iron: Plant-based sources of iron include lentils, beans, tofu, fortified cereals, spinach, and quinoa. Iron from plant sources is less easily absorbed by the body compared to animal-origin iron. To enhance iron absorption, consume iron-rich foods with vitamin C–rich foods, such as citrus fruits, strawberries, or bell peppers.

Calcium: Calcium is essential for developing the baby's bones and teeth. Good plant-based sources of calcium include fortified plant-based milk (like almond or soy), calcium-set tofu, leafy greens (e.g., kale, bok choy), and fortified orange juice.

Vitamin B_{12}: As vitamin B_{12} is primarily found in animal products, it is crucial for pregnant and breastfeeding women following a plant-based diet to take B_{12} supplements or eat B_{12}-enriched foods, like fortified plant-based milk or breakfast cereals.

Folate: Folate (or folic acid) is essential for preventing congenital disabilities. Plant-based sources of folate include leafy greens, legumes, and fortified foods. Folate supplements are also commonly recommended during pregnancy.

Omega-3 fatty acids: Omega-3 fatty acids, especially DHA, are important for the baby's brain and eye development. Abundant plant-based sources of omega-3s include flaxseeds, chia seeds, walnuts, and algal oil supplements.

Iodine: Iodine is necessary for the baby's thyroid function and brain development. Iodized salt and algae (like seaweed) are animal-free sources of iodine.

If necessary, consult a healthcare provider or registered dietitian specializing in prenatal plant-based nutrition. They can assess your specific nutritional needs and provide personalized recommendations.

7. Should I take collagen supplements on a plant-based diet?

Despite the exaggerated benefits of collagen supplementation purported on social media, oral collagen supplements *can* improve skin quality, provide anti-aging benefits, and help manage joint pain caused by osteoarthritis (Miranda et al., 2021; Mobasheri et al., 2021; Woo et al., 2017). Nevertheless, collagen supplements are typically derived from animal sources, such as cows, chickens, or fishes, making them unsuitable for vegans. In fact, collagen is only found in animal tissues like skin, bones, and cartilage, so there is no true plant-based collagen. However, certain nutrients—such as vitamin C, proline, and glycine—support the body's natural collagen production and are often marketed as "plant-based collagen" despite not containing actual collagen.

Plant-based diet benefits: A balanced plant-based diet is rich in antioxidants, vitamins, and minerals that promote healthy skin, hair, nails, and joints. Nutrient-dense foods like fruits, vegetables, nuts, seeds, and whole grains provide the body with essential nutrients that support collagen production and overall skin and joint health.

Vitamin C: Vitamin C is essential for collagen synthesis. Including plenty of vitamin C–rich foods in your diet, such as citrus fruits, berries, kiwi, and bell peppers, can help support collagen production naturally.

Silica-rich foods: Silica is a mineral that plays a role in collagen formation. Foods like oats, brown rice, and leafy greens contain silica and can be included in your diet to support skin and joint health.

Amino acids: Collagen is made up of amino acids, particularly glycine, proline, and hydroxyproline. You can obtain these amino acids from plant-based protein sources, like legumes, tofu, tempeh, quinoa, and plant-based protein powder.

Supplements: If you are concerned about collagen production or have specific skin or joint health issues, you might consider supplements like plant-based amino acid supplements (glycine, proline, or hydroxyproline), biotin, or hyaluronic acid. However, always consult with a healthcare provider or registered dietitian before taking supplements, as they can provide guidance based on your individual needs and health goals.

Collagen-boosting ingredients: Some animal-free ingredients, like seaweed and aloe vera, are claimed to support collagen production and skin health. While research on their effectiveness is limited, including these ingredients in your skin-care routine or diet may be beneficial.

Hydration and sun protection: Staying well hydrated, protecting your skin from excessive sun exposure, and using (vegan-friendly) sun cream are essential for maintaining healthy skin.

In conclusion, you can support your skin and joint health on a plant-based diet by focusing on a nutrient-rich, well-balanced diet that includes foods rich in vitamins, minerals, and amino acids necessary for collagen production.

8. I have diabetes. Can I be vegan?

Yes, individuals with diabetes can follow a vegan diet—and benefit from it. Be mindful that regardless of the diet (omnivore, vegetarian, or vegan), people with diabetes must be careful to manage blood sugar levels effectively. A healthy plant-based diet can improve weight management, boost your energy, stabilize blood sugar levels, and reduce the risk of chronic diseases—including type 1 and type 2 diabetes.

Vegans have up to a 78 percent lower risk of developing type 2 diabetes (Kahleova et al., 2017; Le & Sabaté, 2014). Studies also show that balanced vegan diets can *reverse* type 2 diabetes (Kahleova et al., 2017). Proteins, sugars, growth factors, and hormones (e.g., estrogen) from dairy and meat products activate the secretion of insulin, growth hormone (GH), and insulin-like growth factor (IGF-1), which are associated with type 2 diabetes (Barnard, 2020). Dairy proteins (e.g., β-casein) can also induce immune reactions that destroy pancreatic insulin-producing cells, increasing the risk of type 1 diabetes (Campbell & Campbell II, 2005).

Let's look at some key considerations for people with diabetes who want to adopt a plant-based diet.

Carbohydrate management: Carbohydrates significantly impact blood sugar levels. People with diabetes should focus on consuming complex carbohydrates with a low glycemic index (GI), as they are digested more slowly and have a more gradual effect on blood sugar. Examples of low-GI foods include whole grains (brown rice, quinoa, whole wheat), legumes (beans, lentils), and non-starchy vegetables (leafy greens, broccoli, cauliflower). Avoid refined sugar. Whether it is white sugar, brown sugar, or molasses, they all cause blood sugar peaks.

Portion control: Pay attention to portion sizes to avoid overeating carbohydrates, as even healthy carbohydrates can affect blood sugar if consumed in large quantities.

Fiber intake: Vegan diets tend to be high in fiber, which can help stabilize blood sugar levels. Fiber-rich foods include fruits, vegetables, whole grains, legumes, and nuts.

Protein sources: Include plant-based protein sources like tofu, tempeh, seitan, legumes, and nuts in your diet. Protein can help you feel satisfied and assist with weight management.

Healthy fats: Choose sources of healthy fats (i.e., mono- and poly-unsaturated fats), as they can help improve insulin sensitivity. Good sources of unsaturated fats are avocado, coconut, nuts, seeds, and olive oil. Be careful to consume them in moderation, as fats are high in calories and can cause cardiovascular problems if consumed excessively.

Monitor blood sugar: Regularly monitor your blood sugar levels to understand how different foods and meals affect you. Adjust your diet accordingly in consultation with your healthcare provider.

Consult a registered dietitian: A registered dietitian who specializes in diabetes management and is proficient in plant-based nutrition can provide personalized guidance and meal plans tailored to your specific needs and preferences.

Be mindful of ultra-processed foods: Many overly processed foods, like sugary snacks, ready-to-eat meals, and desserts, can be high in refined carbohydrates and added sugars. Limit your intake of these items.

Stay hydrated: Proper hydration is essential for overall health and can help with blood sugar control.

Regular monitoring and consultation with a healthcare professional are essential for successful diabetes management—on any diet. Also, remember that if you have diabetes, your doctor may need to periodically adjust your medication as your insulin levels improve with a plant-based diet.

9. What are good pre- and post-workout vegan meals?

Sports nutrition plays a crucial role in maximizing the benefits of exercise, promoting recovery, and supporting overall health. Fueling your body properly before and after workouts can help you get the most out of your training and reduce the risk of injury and burnout. Rumor has it that vegans have lower athletic performance and difficulty growing muscle. This is completely false. Many top athletes (including world champions and Olympic weightlifters) are vegan, and plant-based diets are becoming increasingly popular among professional athletes due to their health benefits (Vitale & Hueglin, 2021). Watch the documentaries *Game Changers* and *You Are What You Eat: A Twin Experiment*!

Here are some ideas for pre- and post-workout vegan meals to fuel your exercise, support recovery, and promote muscle growth.

Pre-workout meals (1–2 hours before exercise):

- **Oatmeal**: A bowl of oatmeal topped with sliced bananas, berries, and a sprinkle of nuts or seeds provides complex carbohydrates for sustained energy (and also some protein).

- **Whole-grain toast with nut butter**: Whole-grain toast spread with almond or peanut butter is a good source of carbohydrates and healthy fats. Add sliced banana or a drizzle of maple syrup for extra energy.

- **Avocado toast**: Whole-grain toast spread with avocado is a great source of carbohydrates (for endurance exercises) and healthy fats (for overall health and a more sustained energy source than quickly digested carbohydrates).

- **Smoothie**: Blend a smoothie with plant-based protein powder, spinach or kale, frozen fruit, plant-based milk, and a tablespoon of chia seeds. This provides protein, carbohydrates, and essential nutrients.

- **Quinoa salad**: A quinoa salad with chickpeas, mixed vegetables, and a tahini dressing is rich in protein and complex carbohydrates.

- **Brown rice and tofu**: Brown rice with sautéed tofu, broccoli, and a teriyaki sauce can provide both carbohydrates and protein. This meal is also a great source of calcium and iron.

Post-workout meals (within 1–2 hours after exercise):

- **Protein smoothie**: A smoothie with plant-based protein powder, plant-based milk, a banana, and some spinach is an excellent choice to help repair and build muscle.

- **Chickpea salad**: A salad with chickpeas, mixed greens, cherry tomatoes, cucumber, and tahini-lemon dressing is rich in protein, fiber, and vitamins.

- **Veggie wrap**: Load a whole-grain wrap with hummus, roasted vegetables, and some quinoa for a balanced and protein-rich meal.

- **Tofu stir-fry**: Tofu stir-fried with plenty of vegetables in a soy or teriyaki sauce served over brown rice or quinoa offers both protein and carbohydrates.

- **Sweet potato and bean bowl**: A bowl with roasted sweet potatoes, black beans, salsa, and guacamole combines carbohydrates, high-quality protein, and healthy fats.

- **Hydration is key**: Remember to drink plenty of water before, during, and after your workout to stay hydrated.

- **Snack options**: If you have a smaller gap between your meal and your workout, you can opt for quick snacks like some fruit, a handful of nuts, or a sugar-free granola bar.

- **Timing is important**: Try to time your meals and snacks so that you have enough energy during your workout and can replenish your body's nutrient stores afterward. Adjust your portions and timing based on your workout intensity and goals.

A well-balanced vegan diet can provide all the nutrients for pre- and post-workout nutrition. Focus on a combination of carbohydrates, protein, and unsaturated fats to support energy, recovery, and muscle growth.

10. My partner will not go vegan. What should I do?

In a recent survey, it was found that 56 percent of American vegans would not consider dating one who eats meat (Mridul, 2021). This speaks to the deeply held ideals and convictions that many vegans have regarding animal exploitation, and the potential conflicts that could arise in a relationship with someone who does not share their ethical stance. Asking a vegan if they would date a non-vegan is on par with asking a non-racist if they would date a racist. It is not as much about preference as it is about important core values.

If one wishes to maintain a positive relationship with a non-vegan that is free of or minimizes conflict, it will take flexibility, tolerance, planning, and, above all, communication. Even with people we are close to, we cannot presume to know everything about why they choose the foods they do and engage in activities that contribute to animal oppression. Habits are deeply ingrained, social conformity can be a strong factor, and individuals vary in the degree to which they empathize with others. While you may feel the need to explain to him or her the reasons why you are vegan, it is not wise or productive to become confrontational, criticize them about their diet, or pressure them to change. As a romantic relationship should ultimately be based on mutual love, respect, and caring for each other, keep the focus on why veganism is important to *you*. Active listening is key to understanding where another person is coming from, as are open communication and discussion, where both parties feel secure in expressing their needs and expectations for the relationship.

Here are some practical tips:
- When eating out, research and find restaurants that have both vegan and non-vegan dishes.
- If you are cooking meals together, find recipes that can be adapted to both vegan and non-vegan ingredients.

- Include items in your meal planning that are already vegan—for example, rice, potatoes, breads, and salads.
- In recipes you make for your partner, use some of the many meat alternative products available that are virtually indistinguishable in taste from their animal counterparts. He or she may not even realize that they are eating a vegan dish!
- Bring vegan dishes to social or family gatherings.
- Enjoy snack foods together that are already vegan—for example, popcorn, toast with nut butter, chips and dip, fruit leather, rice cakes, nuts, and hummus with veggies.
- Vegans, in many cases, will use cookware (e.g., pots, pans) reserved for only plant-based cooking, and also refrain from washing items used for meat-based meals.
- Sometimes, an agreement might be reached where partners eat totally vegan while at home, but the non-vegan might order animal products while eating out.

With time, as your partner sees how beneficial and delicious plant-based eating can be, they may come around in their own time and decide to go plant-based. Regarding other aspects of veganism, dialogue and patience remain crucial to help your partner understand the importance of your lifestyle. With a little creativity and adaptability, vegans and non-vegans can learn to enjoy each other's company.

11. I eat meat. Why don't vegans understand my diet is a personal choice?

A common justification for the consumption of animal products is that it is a "personal choice." Behind this reasoning are assumptions that vegans' views are somehow extreme and that they are self-righteous in trying to impose their values on others. Central to this conflict is the social conditioning in which most of us have been raised, where we become disconnected from the larger issues that surround our choices.

When the food we choose to eat involves the suffering and death of another being, it becomes a choice of deeper ethical consequences. Yet it is so easy to "keep the blinders on." We accept a small number of animal species as beloved companions, yet give no thought to harming and consuming others who are no less sentient and feeling.

In truth, most of us in our upbringing did not actually *make* a choice to eat or not eat animals. Rather, we simply accepted what our parents provided for us, as they also did with *their* parents. For most of us, the idea of not consuming animals and animal products never even entered our awareness. However, the times in which we live, with information constantly at our fingertips, give us the opportunity to expand our knowledge, with the realization that the best part of ourselves is our innate empathy and compassion. The personal choices we make every day are opportunities to create a kinder and more just world as we see ourselves in all others. Growing numbers of people are making the shift in awareness, adopting a compassionate lifestyle and refusing to be complicit in the exploitation of the vulnerable.

> We can't plead ignorance, only indifference. Those alive today are the generations that came to know better. [. . .] We are the ones of whom it will be fairly asked, *What did you do when you learned the truth about eating animals?* (Foer, 2009)

12. Don't vegans care about plant suffering?

One of the most common questions that veg-curious people ask is, "Don't plants have feelings?" While it is true that plants react to stimuli, they do not feel pain or emotions. At the cellular level, plants respond to changes in temperature, light, moisture, soil quality, wind, weather, climate, and environmental conditions, and their hormones regulate a wide range of processes, including growth rate, flowering, and seasonal adaptations. Despite the complexities of their sensitivities, plants do not have the physiological substrates and emotional awareness that would enable them to experience pain and suffering. Such an ability depends on having a brain and a nervous system, which plants lack.

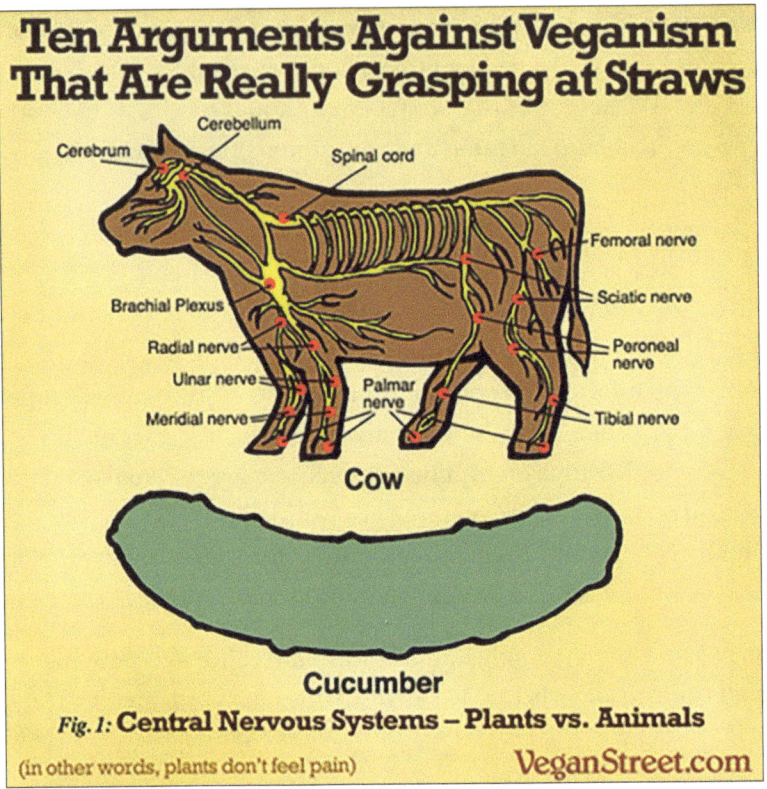

Figure 10. *Central nervous systems—plants vs. animals. Source: VeganStreet.com.*

While animal sentience (as opposed to plant sentience) is exhaustively proven by science, even someone with a primary perception of reality realizes that chopping a carrot is not the same as cutting an animal's head off.

The concern for minimizing harm to living beings and preserving species, including plants, is valid. However, attributing *animal-like* sensations such as pain to plants is not supported by scientific evidence. And, quite frankly, if one is worried about plant suffering, this is more reason to go vegan, as animals feed on plants. Raising animals for food requires much more plant resources than a plant-based diet. This is an established scientific fact.

13. Why do vegans care more about animals than about humans?

That's simply not true. Vegans care about animals because they care about *all* beings. Extending respect to other species doesn't take away from caring for humans. In fact, being vegan is one of the most powerful ways to help other people. From improving overall global health and curbing world hunger to reducing resource depletion, deforestation, pollution, carbon emissions, decimation of our oceans, and biodiversity loss—none of this would be possible without a transformation of our food systems and a worldwide shift to plant-based living. Moreover, by expanding our circle of moral consideration to all sentient lives, we can create a world where non-oppression and justice are taken seriously. All life is interconnected on this planet, and in bringing harm to other sentient beings, we only harm ourselves. Going vegan is about so much more than just diet. It is an opportunity to expand our innate gifts of empathy and compassion and the possibilities for greater peace and sustainability in our lives.

14. Animals eat animals, so why can't I?

Humans are not purely instinctual beings devoid of the capacity to make conscious choices. If we were to justify meat consumption based on other animals' conduct, for consistency, we would have to justify a lot of other behaviors, like copulating with family members and killing each other over territory. There are animals known as obligate carnivores who *must* consume meat to survive. This is a biological necessity enabling them to receive nutrients, such as the amino acid taurine, found only in animal flesh. Examples of obligate carnivores include felines, eagles, snakes, dolphins, and seals. Multiple anatomical, physiological, and behavioral characteristics demonstrate that humans are not strict carnivores.

Numerous comparative studies have shown that the human digestive system and physiology are more suited to consuming plants than to eating animal meat. For example, big cats (lions, cheetahs, tigers) have a large mouth size relative to their heads, and jaws that move only up and down in order to seize and kill prey and swallow meat whole. By contrast, our mouth size is relatively small, with jaws moving both side-to-side and up and down, enabling us to chew and grind vegetation easily. Many meat eaters have sharp, pointed teeth for tearing flesh in a scissor or shear-like motion. By contrast, most herbivores and humans lack these teeth, having flat molars ideal for crushing and grinding plant material. Humans also lack sharp claws and teeth designed for piercing animal skin and tearing muscle tissue. Furthermore, in order to digest animal flesh, the stomach acid of a meat eater's stomach is twenty times stronger than that of a human. We are also uniquely equipped to digest carbohydrates through the enzyme amylase, produced by our salivary glands, and have a substantially longer digestive tract designed to digest the cellulose in plant foods.

These are just a few examples pointing to the relevance of considering physiological capabilities in our dietary choices. It is true that early humans adopted meat-eating because of food availability and survival needs, and most humans today *do function* as omnivores. However, it is *not* a biological necessity for us to consume animals and animal products; at least 70 percent of human diseases are tied to the consumption of animal foods (FAO, 2013).

More and more people are realizing the health benefits of a WFPB diet. Many of the world's top athletes are vegan (as depicted in the 2018 documentary *The Game Changers*), and some of the largest and strongest animals on Earth, such as gorillas, rhinos, and elephants, eat only plants! Moreover, a plant-based food system is a very efficient and *necessary* measure to curb the climate crisis and ensure a decent world for future generations. Because we, as humans, can reason, it is all the more pressing that we use our discerning abilities to make intelligent dietary choices for personal and planetary health. Additionally, our capacities for moral contemplation and ethical reasoning and our ability to thrive on plant-based diets further emphasize the importance of plant-based eating.

15. Do vegans eat eggs from backyard hens?

Vegans do not consume animal products, including eggs. Eating eggs perpetuates the acceptance that animals can be commodified for food, yet the myth persists that it is humane to raise backyard hens. While under ideal conditions backyard hens have a better life than those in industrialized factory farms, the truth remains that chickens are arguably the most exploited animals on the planet—sixty billion killed per year (Whittleton, 2019).

Consumers who purchase hens with good intentions are likely unaware that for every female chicken born, a male is brutally killed through maceration or suffocation, as their breed is unsuitable for meat and they are unable to lay eggs. Furthermore, one is unknowingly supporting the industry as these animals come directly from factory farming facilities. Chickens are the most genetically manipulated animals on the planet, and decades of forced breeding have made current breeds substantially different from their wild counterparts. Chicks often come from large-scale farms specialized in breeding and hatching. During shipping, millions of baby hens die each year due to dehydration, injury, and starvation; in fact, if one orders three birds, twelve are sent with the expectation that nine of them will probably die. Also, it is essential to realize that by *purchasing* animals, we reinforce their property status and support other people in making an earning out of sentient beings.

Raising backyard hens in itself is problematic, even if well-intentioned. There are challenges to maintaining adequate housing, hygiene, food, and socialization, as well as dealing with possible predators, exposure to disease, and the lack of specialized veterinary care. Most people do not realize that egg-laying takes a huge toll on the animals' bodies, including debilitating osteoporosis due to the loss of precious calcium. While it is a practice in some sanctuaries to feed the eggs back to the hens, the nutritional and health concerns of each bird must be taken into consideration (Open Sanctuary Staff, 2018).

There is absolutely no nutritional reason to consume eggs. Eating them is tied to significant health concerns. With high levels of cholesterol and saturated fat, they raise the risk for heart disease, diabetes, and prostate and colorectal cancer (PCRM, undated).

The most compassionate choice we can make as consumers is to simply refuse to use animals.

16. I eat free-range meat and eggs. I'm not hurting animals, am I?

Would you eat free-range *dog* meat? If your answer is no, you already understand the ethical implications of using or killing animals regardless of how they are raised. Sadly, the animal agriculture industry has adopted the term "free range" to suggest that animals are well cared for, conjuring images in consumers' minds of animals living freely in natural outdoor surroundings. Such idyllic depictions have found their way onto product packaging, further instilling the false notion that buyers are making compassionate choices when nothing could be further from the truth.

While the USDA states that so-called free range chicken farms provide access to the outdoors, there are no specific standards stipulating the size of the area or the nature of any ground cover. In many cases, the requirement might be met by a small door allowing access to a muddy strip or concrete floor, an area that might be barely accessible to a few birds out of the many thousands confined in windowless factory farm sheds. Natural behaviors are impossible. Any kind of meaningful regulation is non-existent, and there is no concern for the well-being of the animals outside of commercial interests, for they are seen only as units of production. Cruelty is pervasive in the system, from the hundreds of millions of male chicks suffocated, crushed or ground alive for the simple fact that they cannot produce eggs. Standard industry practices include debeaking, toe-cutting, and slaughter (by throat-slitting) of egg-laying hens at the age of only two once they are no longer productive. Horrific, overcrowded conditions lead to aggressive behaviors and disease. A detailed analysis of the actual meaning of welfare standards and labels is presented in the book *Food for Thought: Planetary Healing Begins on Our Plate* (Perussello, 2022).

Misleading "humane washing" terms are pervasive in marketing labels: "grass fed," "pasture raised," "ethically raised," "high welfare," "humanely raised," "locally sourced," "responsibly sourced," and the list goes on. Consumers are misled to believe they are making ethical food choices, and for the most part remain ignorant of the immense suffering animals endure regardless of whether labelled as "free range" or not. For other farmed animals, industry abuses include dehorning, tail docking, castration, branding, and ear notching, performed without painkillers, and the forcible violation and impregnation of dairy cows restrained with the so-called "rape rack." In one of the cruelest acts of the industry, these cows have their babies taken away from them so their milk can be extracted for human consumption. Numerous practices that cause physical and emotional suffering are *unavoidable* when we use and kill sentient beings, regardless of animal welfare standards. Also, it is astounding when one really thinks about the fact that we are the only animals that continue to consume the milk of another species despite clear evidence that it is harmful to one's health (Mills, 2020).

One of the most significant points of awareness we acquire as vegans is that there is no such thing as humane meat or humane animal by-products. Regardless of how an animal was raised, it will be eventually killed. Our power as consumers is that we can choose *not* to be complicit in the violence and death brought upon our fellow beings. In doing so, we save the lives of animals, and our dedication to living compassionately is a positive and powerful message to put out into the world.

17. I'm vegetarian. I'm not hurting animals, am I?

Unfortunately, vegetarians do hurt animals. Vegetarians certainly are contributing *less* than meat eaters to the suffering and death of billions of animals every year. However, through their continuing consumption of eggs and dairy products, they are subsidizing some of the most cruel practices of the industry, directly tied to the exploitation and abuse of animals, especially females.

The motivations to become vegetarian cover a wide range of concerns, among them animal ethics, the environment, health, economics, food insecurity, and religious, cultural, and social reasons. Currently, there are considerably more vegetarians than vegans globally, and it is not uncommon for many vegans to have first been vegetarian. Donald Watson noted that the word *vegan* is the beginning and the end of the word *vegetarian*. Especially over the past decade, the public has become more knowledgeable and aware of the fundamental differences in the ethical choices between the two. While vegetarians do not eat animal flesh, vegans take it further and also do not consume *any* animal products found in foods, including dairy products (milk, cream, cheese, and yogurt, for example), eggs, and honey. They also avoid, to the greatest extent possible, using products that contain animal-derived ingredients and those that have been tested on animals. As noted earlier in this book, animal products are found in a wide range of items: clothing and accessories, cosmetics, lotions, shampoos, medicines, supplements, cleaning materials, and furnishings. Additionally, ethical vegans do not support any activity that involves animal use, imprisonment, suffering, and oppression, like zoos and horse riding.

Using animals implies inflicting unnecessary suffering on them, *regardless* of the production method. Moreover, blatantly cruel practices are common and, many times, *inevitable* in animal farming. Hens suffer the painful procedure of having part of their beaks seared off, without anesthesia, in order to reduce aggression and cannibalism during confinement in battery cages. Five to eleven birds are crammed together in a single cage so small they are unable to even spread their wings. The level of suffering is severe: feces and urine falling through the stacked cages; injuries caused by constant friction with cage wires; skeletal disorders, osteoporosis and broken bones from constant calcium depletion; periods where food and water are withheld to force higher egg production; prolapse, a common condition where the ovaries and uterus eject during egg-laying, causing an agonizing death; and intense psychological, traumatic stress. In these miserable conditions, hens rarely live past two years, and are then sent to slaughter. While some countries have banned or are phasing out battery cages, in the United States, three-fourths of hens are raised in states without cage regulations (USDA, 2023). And it's not only the females that suffer. Because male chicks of this breed are unsuited for meat, they are ground up alive in macerators, gassed, or suffocated. In the United States, over 200 million of them are killed every year. These innocent baby chicks are nothing but disposable units to the egg industry. They are born to be killed.

Dairy cows are restrained and forcibly impregnated in what is known as a "rape rack." Newborn calves are taken away from their mothers; the males, since they cannot produce milk, are either killed or confined in crates to be raised for veal. While the average natural lifespan of a cow is fifteen to twenty years, most cows raised for milk are slaughtered after only four to five years, their bodies spent from enduring repeated impregnation and forced milk production hooked up to machines. In many instances, they become lame and infected with mastitis, a painful and highly contagious inflammatory disease. As animal rights advocate and Rutgers University law professor Gary Francione states, "There is probably more suffering in a glass of milk or an ice cream cone than there is in a steak" (Francione, undated).

There is no denying that the egg and dairy industries are immensely and gruesomely cruel. While advertisements and marketing images mislead customers into believing there are "ethical" egg and dairy products, in this day and age, it is easy to educate ourselves and learn the truth. Being vegetarian is a start, but by ultimately adopting a vegan lifestyle, we fully commit to our compassionate values by refusing to exploit the innocent and the vulnerable.

18. Isn't eating local more important than eating plant-based to reduce your carbon footprint?

Plant-based diets have a significantly lower carbon footprint than others. A vegan diet emits up to 73 percent less greenhouse gases (GHGs) than an omnivore diet (Poore & Nemecek, 2018; Ritchie, 2020). That is because carbon emissions from transportation and processing represent a tiny fraction of food production emissions, especially for animal products (Figure 11). For instance, consuming locally grown, seasonal produce within a plant-based diet can be a good choice for reducing transportation-related emissions—but if you are eating locally sourced meat or dairy, these will have a significantly higher carbon footprint than plant-based proteins.

What we eat (plant versus animal foods) is far more important than *where* the food traveled from. This has been proven time and time again (Clark & Tilman, 2017; Poore & Nemecek, 2018; Ritchie, 2020; Hayek et al., 2020). If we can create a plant-based food system *and* encourage local consumption, this is definitely a plus.

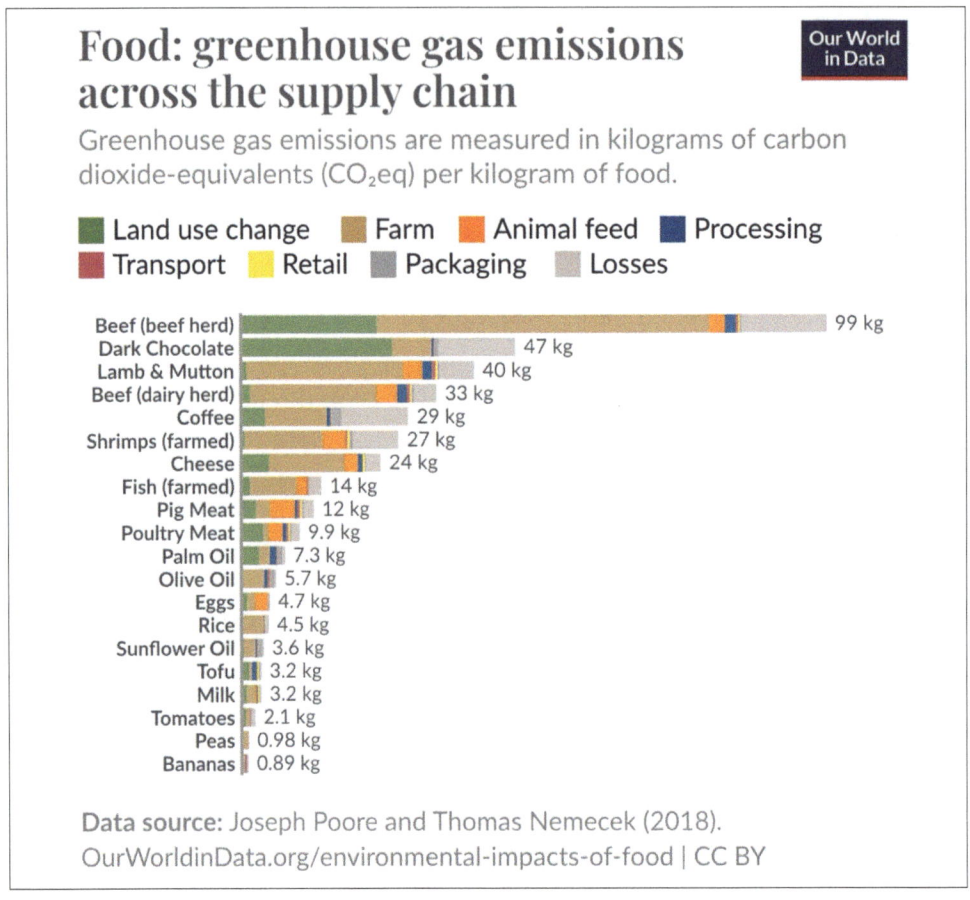

Figure 11. *Carbon emissions across the food supply chain. Source: Ritchie (2020).*

The "local eating" argument is a common misconception used to dismiss the importance of plant-based eating. Although the carbon footprint of different products depends on various factors, including place of origin, eating local animal products is not as environmentally beneficial as eating a plant-based diet. The exception would be extreme cases; for example, an isolated community in Alaska or Siberia that has abundant fish sources but poor access to plant-origin foods. These are rare exceptions that do not reflect the reality of most people.

The livestock industry is a major contributor to GHG emissions due to deforestation and ruminant animal metabolism. Contrary to popular belief, seafood consumption is also linked to deforestation and carbon emissions, as farmed water animals are fed crops. Moreover, lower carbon emissions are not the only environmental benefit of ditching animal products. Plant-based diets significantly reduce land, air, and water pollution, preserving soil, forests, and oceans and thereby protecting our planet's biodiversity. The omnivore diet, in turn, is associated with higher water and land use, species extinction, antibiotic resistance, and a range of animal-origin diseases.

In summary, eating both plant-based and local can lower one's carbon footprint while supporting local economies and potentially sustainable farming practices, like veganic agriculture (VAN, 2022). A combination of both strategies, where you eat exclusively plant foods and prioritize locally sourced items, would be the ideal scenario. Additionally, other factors like reducing food waste, choosing organic foods, and minimizing packaging can further reduce the environmental impact of your diet.

19. What will happen to animal farmers if we all go vegan?

Oftentimes, people will ask this question as if the whole world would suddenly become vegan overnight, like the flipping of a light switch. However, such a broad-scale change would happen slowly over a period of time, as consumer demand for animal products declines, accompanied by a reduction in the number of animals killed for food. Consumer choices due to health, environmental, and ethical considerations are driving the plant-based food market and a transformative shift in food production, with more and more farmers switching to growing plants. These are just a few examples:

- Bob Comis, the subject of Allison Argo's touching documentary *The Last Pig* (2017), faced a crisis in compassionate awareness, giving up his work as a livestock farmer to grow vegetables instead.
- The website Free From Harm (www.freefromharm.org) profiles the rising numbers of farmers who have transitioned to growing plant foods.

- Dairy milk consumption has declined 42 percent from fifty years ago (CBS News, 2022), with the number of US dairy farms falling by more than 50 percent between 1997 and 2017 (Lakhani, 2023).
- Companies such as Elmhurst Dairy, New York state's largest dairy, closed in 2016 due to declining sales, then reopened in 2017 as a producer of only plant-based milks under the motto, MISSION TRANSLATION: CHANGE YOUR DIET. CHANGE THE WORLD.
- More and more organizations are assisting farmers to make the shift, such as Mercy For Animals' project called *Transfarmation*: www.thetransfarmationproject.org/.

Awareness of the damages of animal agriculture is driving a shift in the food landscape toward plant-based eating. However, farmers making the transition away from livestock farming is only part of the solution. As you will read in FAQ #20, fundamental, systemic changes are critically needed, as a hugely disproportionate amount of government funding currently supports and subsidizes the meat and dairy industries. Ultimately, as a society, we must question how we can continue enabling industries that bring such horrific cruelty and death to innocent, sentient beings.

20. Animal agriculture contributes significantly to the GDP of most nations. Is a plant-based food system economically feasible?

The fact that a sector is profitable does not mean it remains morally justifiable throughout the centuries. As the world's moral code evolves, fewer of us support industries and livelihoods that are highly lucrative but hurt others. There are many examples of that around us. That said, transitioning to a plant-based food system is economically feasible with the proper adaptation of the existing agricultural and economic structures.

Obviously, the transition would not happen overnight, leaving people jobless. In fact, the transition is *already happening* in incremental steps. Ever more farms and companies are switching to plant-sourced foods, as explained in FAQ #19. Animal farmers have been transitioning to growing crops for many reasons, including economic issues and ethical considerations. For example, a 2022 survey by the Irish Farmers Association revealed that 80 percent of producers would not recommend this career for younger generations (Ryan, 2022).

Here are some key points to consider regarding the economic viability of a plant-based food system:

Animal-sourced Foods are Highly Subsidized:

Animal agriculture does contribute significantly to the gross domestic product (GDP) of many nations, and it has created a complex network of jobs, industries, and economic activities. However, the animal exploitation industry is deeply integrated into the global economy thanks to massive public funding, as noted here:

> Animal agriculture is not regulated by free supply and demand. Federal subsidies, tax breaks, corporate grants, and insurance policies created a fail-proof food system where the livestock sector is protected regardless of reductions in market demand. US taxpayers pay USD 38 *billion* in direct and indirect subsidies every year for the killing of animals and environmental destruction—even when they are vegan. Conversely, subsidies towards fruits and vegetables total USD 17 *million*. (Perussello, 2020)

A recent study (Vallone & Lambin, 2023) discusses how public and private investment artificially delays food system transformation (Figure 12). Governments continue funding animal farming through a variety of support mechanisms, dismissing the enormous climate- and disease-mitigation power of whole plant foods and alternative proteins. The study analyzed the main agricultural policies in the EU and the United States in 2014–2020. It revealed that plant-based alternatives received only 0.1 percent of the money spent on meat and dairy:

> In the EU, cattle farmers got at least 50% of their income from direct subsidies. [. . .] For research and innovation spending, 97% went to animal farmers, with almost all of these funds aimed at improving production. (Vallone & Lambin, 2023)

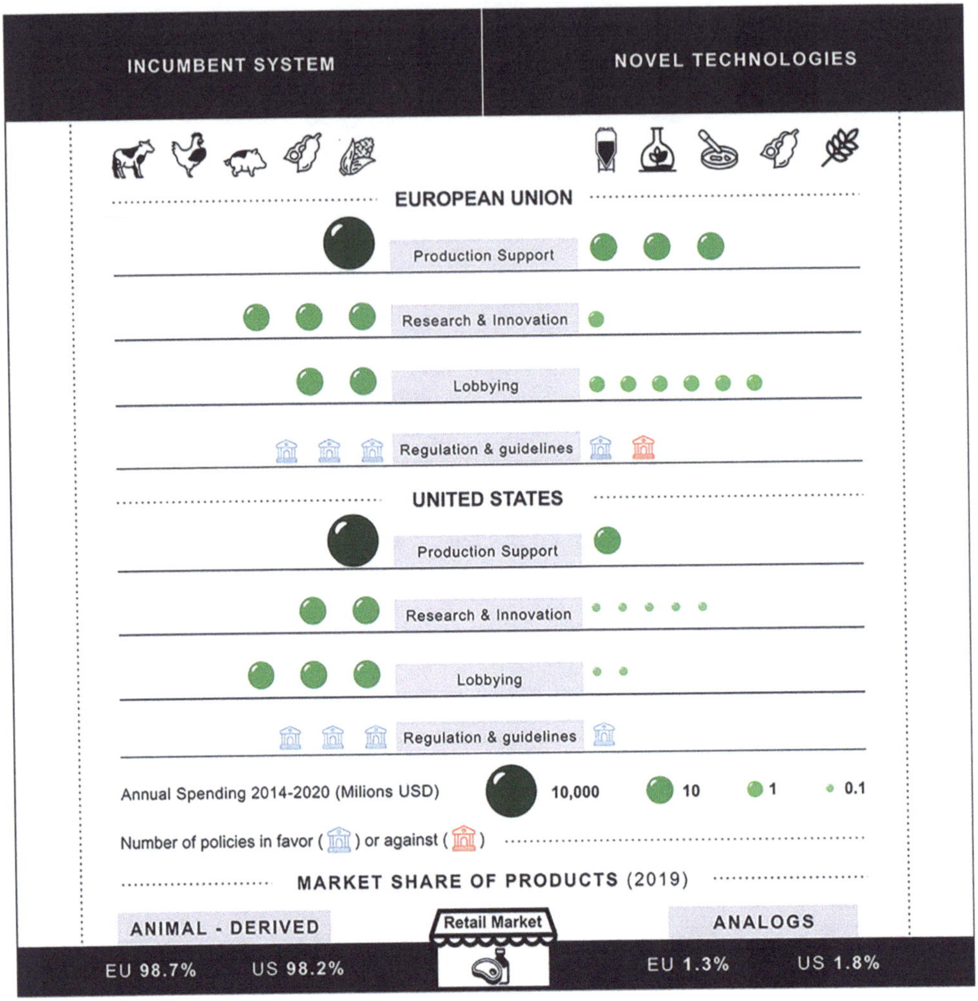

Figure 12. *Public investment in food production: animal-origin foods versus alternatives. Source: Vallone & Lambin (2023).*

The dairy industry has been facing a financial crisis for decades. State subsidies in many countries have artificially made milk prices lower than production costs. Massive investment aims to boost internal consumption and open export markets to help the sector stay afloat (Simon, 2013; Perussello, 2022). The egg and fish sectors also rely on public funding. In the EU, the Common Agricultural Policy (CAP) provides direct payments to farmers based on the size of their land and the number of animals they keep. The USDA provides grants and loans to egg producers for research, education, marketing, and infrastructure development. Globally, USD 15–35 billion of public money is directed to the fish industry (UNEP, 2008).

Transition Challenges and Opportunities:

EU and US livestock farmers receive about 1,000 times more public funding than plant-based and cultivated meat (Carrington, 2023; Vallone & Lambin, 2023). A just transition will mean financial incentives flow in the right direction. Governments can play a crucial role in facilitating food system change by implementing supportive policies and providing investment to ensure a fair transition for those affected.

Financial support can be diverted from meat, dairy, fish, honey, and eggs to farmers who grow plants, algae, and mushrooms. With the help of engineers, their equipment can be retrofitted or simply repurposed. For instance, dairy processing equipment can be used for plant-milk processing. Additionally, animal farmers' and businesses' know-how and existing supply chains can be used to kickstart their new occupations.

Crop farming, innovative protein sources, and plant-based food industries have shown growth potential and can create new and unforeseen economic opportunities. Investing in research and development for plant agriculture, vertical farms, veganic permaculture, plant-based technologies, precision fermentation, and food processing engineering can stimulate economic activity and new occupational branches.

Healthcare and Environmental Savings:

Transitioning to a plant-based diet can provide long-term economic benefits by reducing healthcare costs and premature deaths associated with undernutrition and diseases linked to animal product consumption. As discussed in other chapters, food insecurity is closely tied to animal-origin foods due to resource overuse. Additionally, the environmental impact of animal agriculture, such as GHG emissions and deforestation, imposes economic costs and affects livelihoods, especially in vulnerable communities. Shifting to a more sustainable food system could mitigate these costs. Recent studies show that the transition could bring over USD 10 trillion worth of benefits annually (FAO, 2023).

Food Innovation and Consumer Research:

Increasing consumer demand for plant-based products is already driving changes in the market. As consumer preferences shift, businesses are adapting to meet this demand, creating economic opportunities in the plant-based sector. Investment in food engineering research focused on plants and cellular agriculture ingredients can help maximize resource use, expand current possibilities, and feed the planet tasty, diverse, and healthier food. Also, investment in consumer behavior research can help us better understand consumer needs and preferences and translate this into a wider offer of healthy and appealing products.

Encouraging investment in consumer education is also essential to build a more transparent food system where people are empowered to make informed food choices.

Social Justice:

A global plant-plant food system would be a major social justice accomplishment. Using animals normalizes violence and oppression of the vulnerable. If we can create a world where fellow sentient creatures are not exploited and killed by the billions every year, we can advance a society aligned with values of justice, peace, and non-harm.

In summary, while transitioning to a plant-based food system may pose financial challenges initially, it is feasible with the right policies, incentives, and investments. The long-term benefits (environmental, health, social, economic) make it an unmissable opportunity.

21. What are some tips for traveling as a vegan?

Traveling as a vegan has become much easier over the years, with a wide range of resources available to help you plan your trips in advance. Here are some tips:

- No matter where you are traveling around the world, Happy Cow (www.happycow.net) is a terrific resource (there is also an app available for download). It lists vegan and vegetarian restaurants, including reviews; mentions establishments with vegan options; and gives a rundown of vegan-friendly hotels, bed-and-breakfasts, resorts, stores carrying vegan items, as well as local organizations and community groups devoted to veganism. There is also a chat board, blogs covering a wide variety of articles, and even an online vegan store.
- There are numerous travel blogs about being vegan in destinations around the world, such as The Nomadic Vegan (www.thenomadicvegan.com) and Vegan Travel (www.vegantravel.com). Once arriving at your destination, talk to local folks to get the inside scoop on the best vegan-friendly restaurants and grocery stores. Support local vegan restaurants while traveling.
- Fortunately, many restaurants now offer vegan options. Also, ethnic restaurants, such as Chinese, Thai, Ethiopian, and Indian, often have dishes that are traditionally vegan, but you should not hesitate to ask the waiter to check with the chefs. Restaurants are ideal places to educate others about what vegan means! Though not always the healthiest, even some fast-food establishments now offer vegan items.
- Websites such as Vegvisits (www.vegvisits.com) and VeggieHotels (www.veggie-hotels.com) make it easy to search for vegan accommodations.
- When booking a regular hotel, it is worth doing a map search for nearby grocery stores and restaurants with vegan options. For example, see if a Whole Foods Market is within walking distance. You may also find out if a farmers' market is taking place during your stay.
- Ideally, your hotel room should at least have a microwave and, if possible, a mini-fridge.

- It is a good idea to check out in advance what kind of breakfast options are available where you are staying.
- Staying at a vegan Airbnb is another option, especially if a kitchen is available for you to do your own cooking!
- At restaurants, don't be afraid to ask if a dish can be "veganized" or if a vegan dish can be made especially for you. In some cases, you may need to create a vegan meal by combining side dishes or appetizers.
- In the event that you will be a guest in someone's home, be sure to let them know in advance that you eat plant-based, and maybe offer to do some of the cooking!
- See if there are any local vegan meetups in the city you are visiting.
- In case you are unable to get to a store or restaurant, more and more vegan meal delivery services are popping up, such as Vegan Xpress (www.veganexpressaz.com) and Purple Carrot (www.purplecarrot.com). One can also use services like Uber Eats (www.ubereats.com), Grubhub (www.grubhub.com), and DoorDash (www.doordash.com) to order meals from local restaurants with vegan options.
- For road trips, cooler bags with ice packs can be used as needed, but there are many options for non-perishable vegan snacks too: nuts and seeds, trail mix, energy or snack bars, chips, crackers, fresh fruits, dried fruits, and vegan jerky.
- Air travel presents particular challenges. While many domestic flights have reduced their meal services, many major airlines provide complete vegan meals for long international trips. Be sure to make the request when you book your ticket, and it doesn't hurt to call the airline within a week of travel to be sure your meal is confirmed. The labeling of meals varies from airline to airline; some will use the word *vegan*, while others use names like *strict vegetarian*, so research this carefully. The plus side of eating vegan on these flights is that you will oftentimes be served first! However, eating vegan in airline terminals can be especially difficult, on top of expensive airport prices. Ethnic, "health food," and even fast-food eateries may be possibilities. In the United States, VeggL (www.veggl.com) lists vegan options in a number of airports. Overall,

airports are behind when it comes to meeting vegans' needs. Your best, most affordable option may be to bring food items with you in your carry-on bag to eat during a layover. This can be a little tricky—one can bring in whole fruits, but the amount of any sauces, dips, spreads, jams, dressings, or condiments cannot exceed 100 g each.

- The discussion website Reddit can be a great place for information and ideas. A popular topic is r/Vegan Travel. Tripadvisor is another good resource.
- One of the challenges of foreign travel is asking about food ingredients in restaurants. The Vegan Passport app and V-Cards (www.maxlearning.net/HEALth/V-Cards.pdf) provide phrases in different languages. One can even use Google Translate to assist with instant translations on the spot as you are having a conversation.
- More and more vegan cruises, tours, and vacation packages are available, such as Vegan Cruises (www.vegan-cruises.com) and Responsible Travel (www.responsiblevacation.com/vacations/vegan).

22. It's impossible to be 100 percent vegan, so why even try?

There is a well-known aphorism, "Don't let the perfect be the enemy of the good." Going vegan is not about achieving an objectively defined, absolute point of "perfection." Rather, the goal is to make choices, to the largest extent possible and practical, that align with our values and priorities, among them personal health, environmental sustainability, justice, and respect for animals.

As consumers, it is impossible to know all the instances where our daily lives intersect with animal exploitation. In achieving maximum economic profit in an industry that sees animals solely as production units, animal agriculture commodifies as much of an animal's body as possible, in ways that may not be apparent to the consumer. For example, animal fat may be found in a wide range of products such as asphalt, car tires, caulking compounds, drywall, cement, cosmetics, deodorants, paints, polishes, perfumes, detergents, plastic bags, printer ink, lubricants, soaps, candles, and many more.

While it may not be possible to be 100 percent vegan, we can aspire to make conscious decisions that avoid and minimize the exploitation of animals. For many vegans, there is peace of mind and an expanded sense of compassion that comes from not ingesting and wearing the body parts of a once sentient, feeling being. Shankar Narayan, a well-known vegan advocate in India, has this wonderful saying: "Veganism is not a destination; it is a journey." We cannot eliminate *all* animal products in our daily lives, but we can continue to make choices that celebrate peaceful living.

Chapter 6

Recipes

In this chapter, we compiled a diverse selection of recipes from vegan contributors with varied lifestyles and professional backgrounds living in different parts of the world. Our common bond is a love for animals and great food! Our goal is to demonstrate how easy, healthy, and delicious plant-based eating can be, regardless of your cultural identity, cooking experience, or what you do for a living.

Below, you will find categorized recipes for easy reference. Additionally, brief biographies of the recipe contributors are provided so you get to know a little bit about us. Enjoy!

Our Recipes

Breakfast	Main Dishes	Sauces & Sides	Soups & Breads	Salads & Sandwiches	Desserts
Healthy Oatmeal with Fruit	Miso-Glazed Tofu with Vegetables	Tortilla Chips	Kale & Quinoa Soup	Watermelon Salad	Irresistible Chocolate Mousse
Tofu Scramble on Sourdough	Veggie Wrap with Quinoa Crepes	Mango Salsa	Spicy Brown Lentil Soup with Sour Cream	Mediterranean Chickpea Salad Sandwich	Sweet Cherry Ice Cream with Chocolate Sauce
French Toast Bake	Easy but Delicious Chili	Algarvian Guacamole	Focaccia al Rosmarino	Rainbow Salad	Baked Banana
Sweet or Savory Buckwheat Crepes	Pasta Carbonara	Asparagus with Hollandaise Sauce	Creamy Mushroom Soup with Savory Cashew Cream	Crunchy Tempeh Salad	Coconut Kisses
	Vegetable & Tempeh Wellington with Shiitake Gravy	Homemade Cucumber Pickles	Yummy Spelt Bread	Chickpea & Artichoke Salad	Oatmeal Walnut Cookies
	Hearts of Palm Pie	Simple Marinara Sauce		Crispy Sweet & Sour Tempeh Sourdough Sandwich	Blueberry & Banana Muffins
	Refried Bean Tacos with Caramelized Plantains			Chef AJ's House Salad	Lemon Tofu Mousse

	Ramen Bowl with Fresh Daikon & Greens				Mini Chocolate Orange Cups
	Instant Pot-Atouille				
	Linguine with Artichoke Hearts				
	Feijoada (Brazilian Bean Stew)				
	Portobello Mushroom Stroganoff				
	Chipotle Bean Burgers				

Recipe Contributors

NANCY ARENAS

Nancy is a certified vegan nutrition coach, vegan chef, and founder and organizer of the Red & Green VegFest in Albuquerque, New Mexico. She publishes the magazine *New Mexico Vegan* and runs the non-profit *Sprouting Compassion* and the podcast *Vegan Pulse*. Nancy is an active speaker and advocate for the vegan lifestyle.

CHEF AJ

Chef AJ has been devoted to a plant-exclusive diet for over forty-six years. A chef, culinary instructor, and professional speaker, she is the author of three bestselling books (*The Secrets to Ultimate Weight Loss: A Revolutionary Approach to Conquer Cravings, Overcome Food Addiction and Lose Weight Without Going Hungry*; *Own Your Health*; and the 10th Anniversary Edition of *Unprocessed*), all of which have received glowing endorsement by many luminaries in the plant-based movement. She broadcasts *CHEF AJ LIVE!* on YouTube, Facebook, Instagram, and X, formerly known as Twitter, daily. In 2018, she was inducted into the Vegetarian Hall of Fame.

FERNANDO GRANDO

Fernando is a mechanical engineer with a PhD in tribology and an international career in Formula 1. In his free time, he enjoys creating simple yet tasty vegan meals. When telling how he loves to zip through grocery aisles looking for new plant-based ingredients, he jokes that his true calling is raising the demand for vegan products. Buckle up because Fernando's culinary creations are a high-speed adventure for your taste buds!

JOANNE KONG

Joanne, this book's co-author, is a classical pianist and university lecturer. For her, being vegan touches upon so much more than creating tasty and nutritious dishes. Becoming plant-based has enhanced her mental clarity and empathy and helped her realize deeper inner peace and spirituality. It also expanded her openness to seeing that all beings are connected. Websites: www.vegansmakeadifference.com and www.joannekongmusic.com.

JIM McGEHEE

Jim is a retired chemical research engineer based in Houston, Texas. He loves to cook simple dishes and enjoys the abundance of spices and specialty foods from around the world, which make vegan cooking delicious. The emerging podcast community with potlucks gives him plenty of practice!

KAROLINE MUELLER

Karoline believes that life feels better and more vibrant with good, healthy food. In 2015, she became a Food for Life instructor with the Physicians Committee for Responsible Medicine, and she now teaches healthy vegan cooking classes.

CAMILA PERUSSELLO

Camila, this book's co-author, is a food engineer and researcher. Her home cooking combines Brazilian, Italian, and Portuguese flavors, reflecting her diverse cultural heritage. As a true foodie, she embraces the opportunity to explore new dishes and ingredients wherever she goes. Her passion for food, nature, and traveling the world infuses her cooking with rich flavors (and a touch of adventure!). Website: www.camilaperussello.com.

NANCY POZNAK

Nancy Poznak is a health educator and founder of *BotaniCuisine: Plant-Sourced Dining Outreach*, in Baltimore, Maryland. She has hosted numerous events focused on plant-based vegan outreach, education, and social interactions. She opened Wild Heart Bistro, which serves delicious, entirely plant-sourced foods that appeal to everyone, and provides outreach materials.

CHRISTOPH WAGNER

A passionate advocate for plant-based nutrition and sustainability, Christoph is a certified nutrition coach and personal trainer through the National Academy of Sports Medicine. He also holds a certificate in plant-based nutrition from Cornell University through the T. Colin Campbell Center for Nutrition Studies. An acclaimed classical cellist, he and Joanne Kong have formed *Vegan Virtuosi*, using the power of music to advocate for a more compassionate world.

MARLENE WATSON-TARA

Marlene is a vegan advocate and high-profile chef. She has spent decades training chefs for royal families, world business leaders, and people from the world of music and arts. Her studies and teaching of traditional Chinese medicine and macrobiotics for the past forty years have given her the skills to create bold flavors using the five tastes. She kindly contributed delightful recipes from her book *Go Vegan* (Lotus Publishing, 2019). Websites: www.macrovegan.org and www.humanecologyproject.com.

6.1 Breakfast

Healthy Oatmeal with Fruit
Recipe by Joanne Kong

Ingredients

- 3/4 cup quick-cooking rolled oats
- 1 cup plant-based milk
- 1/2 banana, sliced
- Small apple, chopped
- Fresh or freeze-dried blueberries or strawberries
- 1/4 cup chopped walnuts
- 1/8 tsp cinnamon
- Optional: 2 Tbsp of canned beans or nut butter

Instructions

1. In a deep bowl, mix oatmeal and plant-based milk.
2. Cook in the microwave on high for 1½ to 2 minutes.
3. Mix the remaining ingredients, adding extra milk and heating as needed for desired consistency.

Note: Mix and match fruits, nuts, seeds, and spices for different versions of this recipe!

Recipes

153

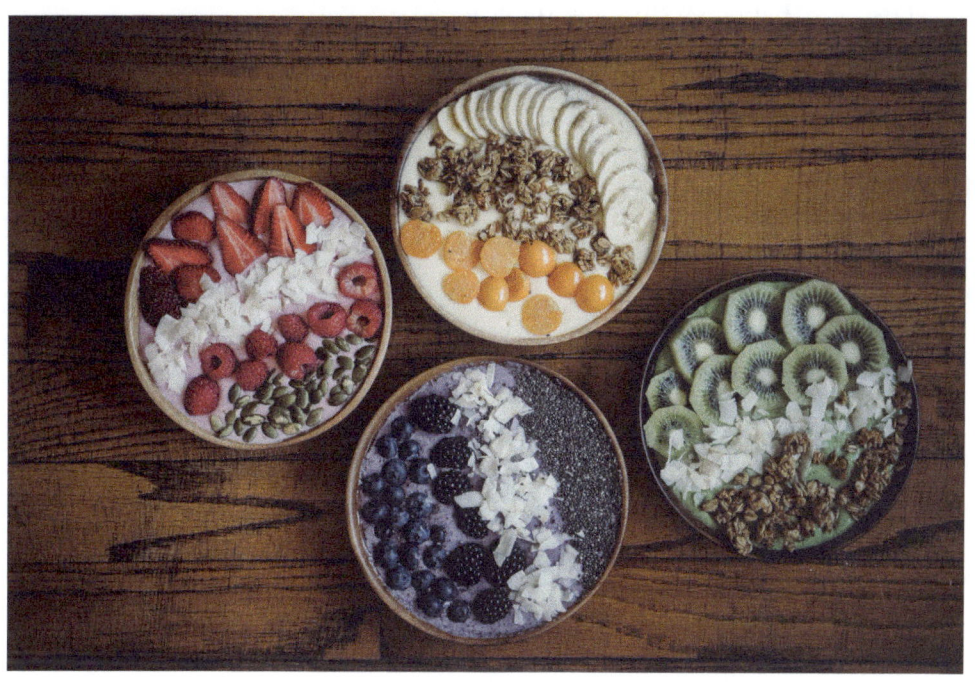

Photo credit: Nicola Barts (www.pexels.com).

Tofu Scramble on Sourdough

Recipe by Marlene Watson-Tara

Ingredients
- 2 shallots, thinly sliced
- 1/2 tsp turmeric
- 1 sweet red pepper, diced
- 60 g (2 oz) button mushrooms, thinly sliced
- 3 spring onions, thinly sliced on the diagonal
- 150 g (5 oz) sweet corn
- 1 pack organic silken tofu
- 1 Tbsp shoyu
- 125 mL (1/2 cup) water
- 1 sheet nori seaweed, cut into small threads
- Handful coriander, chopped
- 1 Tbsp toasted black sesame seeds
- Parsley, minced for garnish

For the tahini sauce:
- 2 Tbsp tahini
- 1 Tbsp shoyu
- 1 clove garlic
- 1 tsp Dijon mustard
- 3 Tbsp nutritional yeast
- 125 (1/2 cup) mL water

Instructions
1. In a high-speed blender, blend the tahini, garlic, mustard, nutritional yeast, and water. Set it aside.
2. In a heavy-based pan, warm a splash or two of water over medium heat. Add the shallots and turmeric, cover, and allow to sweat for 5 minutes.
3. Add the red pepper, mushrooms, spring onions, and corn. Sauté for a further 5–8 minutes.

4. Crumble or mash the tofu into the pan and add the shoyu along with the water. Cover and cook for 5 minutes.
5. Stir in the creamy tahini mixture, nori threads, and coriander. Stir well and remove from the heat.
6. Sprinkle with the black sesame seeds and garnish with parsley. Serve hot piled high on some toasted sourdough or a crusty whole-grain baguette.

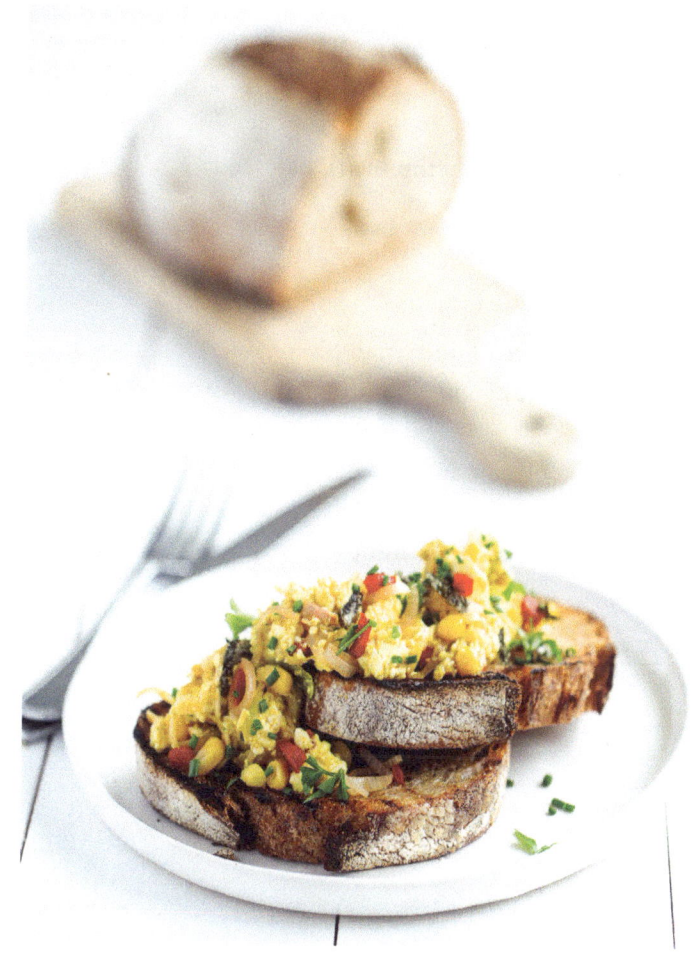

Source: Go Vegan (Lotus Publishing, 2019).

French Toast Bake
Recipe by Nancy Arenas

Ingredients
- Bread (6–8 slices)
- Cinnamon
- Vegan butter
- Maple syrup
- 125 mL (1/2 cup) orange juice
- 125 mL (1/2 cup) plant-based milk
- Vanilla
- Optional add-ins: chia seeds, hemp seeds, flax seeds

Instructions
1. Toast the bread slightly.
2. Add a dab of butter to the baking dish.
3. In a bowl, break up the bread into small pieces.
4. Mix in the cinnamon, orange juice, milk, maple syrup, and vanilla. Adjust to preferred moistness.
5. Mix well, then put the mixture into the baking dish (in a thin layer). Place three dabs of butter on top.
6. Bake at 218°C (425°F) for 15–20 minutes, turning the baking dish halfway through.

Sweet or Savory Buckwheat Crepes
Recipe by Marlene Watson-Tara

Ingredients
For the dough
- 90 g (3/4 cup) buckwheat flour
- 90 g (3/4 cup) unbleached white flour
- 2 tsp baking powder
- 2 small ripe bananas, chopped
- 1 1/2 cups oat or soy milk
- 1/2 cup sparkling water
- 1 Tbsp apple cider vinegar
- Filtered water as desired

For the filling
A. Savory filling:
    - 2 garlic cloves
    - 2 onions
    - 12 chestnut mushrooms
    - 1 red or yellow pepper
    - 1 courgette
    - Tamari
    - 1/2 cup coriander or parsley, chopped
    - Pesto
    - Mayonnaise
B. Sweet filling:
    - Banana
    - Fresh berries
    - Date, maple, or brown rice syrup

Instructions

For the dough

1. Mix the dry ingredients in a large bowl.
2. Place the bananas and wet ingredients in a high-speed blender. Blend along with the dry ingredients to create a smooth mixture.
3. Heat a crepe maker, flat pan, or griddle to a high heat. Pour on half a cup of the mixture and spread with a crepe spreader. Cook the crepe for 2–3 minutes. Bubbles will form and the edges will brown.
4. Carefully push a spatula under the edge of the crepe all the way around. Flip and cook for another few minutes on the other side.

Makes 6 large crepes.

Note: If you prefer a thinner crepe, add more water to the mixture. Use other flours, such as whole-wheat pastry flour, or mix the quantities. When blueberries are in season, I add a half-cup to the mixture.

For the filling

A. Savory version:
   1. Mince the garlic and cut all the vegetables into small dice.
   2. Warm a splash or two of filtered water in a heavy-based pan. Sauté the garlic and onion for 5 minutes.
   3. Add the vegetables and a splash or two of tamari. Cover and cook for 10 minutes, stirring occasionally and adding more water if the pan seems dry.
   4. Stir in the fresh herbs and transfer the vegetables to a covered dish.
   5. When the crepe is warm, spread it with some basil, watercress pesto, and vegan mayonnaise.
   6. Add the roasted vegetables and roll or fold the crepes in half. These savory crepes go great with a warm bowl of soup.

B. Sweet version:
   1. Slice the bananas and add all fruits and syrup to the warm crepes. Roll or fold the crepes in half.

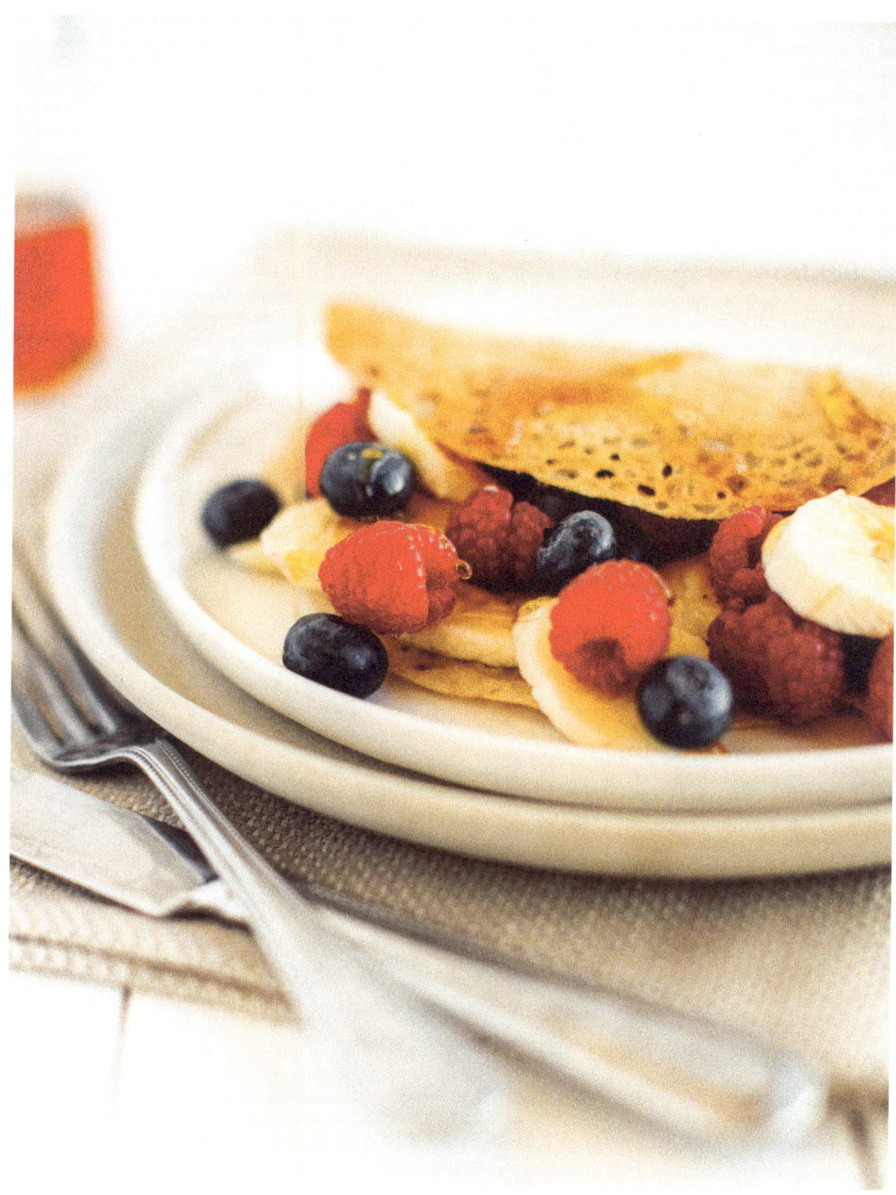

Source: *Go Vegan (Lotus Publishing, 2019).*

6.2 Main Dishes

Miso-Glazed Tofu with Veggies
Recipe by Joanne Kong

Ingredients
- 1 Tbsp white miso
- 1 Tbsp balsamic vinegar
- 1 Tbsp Bragg® liquid aminos
- 1 1/2 Tbsp date syrup
- 2 Tbsp water
- Vegetable broth
- Large clove of garlic, peeled and finely chopped
- 450 g (16 oz) extra-firm tofu, cut into chunks
- 1/2 medium onion, chopped
- 1/2 red bell pepper, seeded and sliced
- 1 cup broccoli florets
- 1/2 cup chopped walnuts or cashews
- Optional: 1 cup frozen pineapple or mango chunks, defrosted

Instructions
1. Using a small whisk, make the sauce by combining the miso, vinegar, liquid aminos, date syrup, and water.
2. In a pan, sauté the garlic in 2 Tbsp of vegetable broth until slightly browned.
3. Add tofu and cook until one side is lightly browned. Flip pieces, add half of the sauce, and cook for 2 or 3 more minutes.
4. Add the remaining ingredients and the rest of the sauce, and continue to cook until heated through. Add additional vegetable broth as needed.

Makes 2 servings.

Veggie Wrap with Quinoa Crepes
Recipe by Karoline Muller

Ingredients

For the crepes
- 2 cups quinoa
- 1/2 tsp salt
- 1 tsp baking powder, or 1/2 tsp baking soda and 1/2 tsp cream of tartar
- 1 cup water
- Oil as needed

For the filling
- 1/4 cup hummus or 1/4 avocado per crepe/wrap
- Veggie ideas:
    - Lettuce leaves
    - Carrot, thinly sliced
    - Cucumber strips
    - Bell pepper strips
    - Onion, sliced
    - Pickles, sliced
    - Olives, sliced
    - Sprouts

Instructions

For the crepes
1. Wash the quinoa well, swirling and rinsing with water several times through a strainer. Place all the quinoa in a covered bowl with plenty of water and let it soak for at least 6 hours.
2. Wash and swirl again to remove all foam. Using the strainer, transfer all the quinoa to the blender jar.

3. Add 1 cup of water, or until the level reaches 1 quart (approximately 950 g). Blend well. Add salt and baking powder (or baking soda and cream of tartar). Blend again.
4. Heat crepe pan or griddle. Using oil as needed, ladle approximately 50 g of batter onto the hot surface and spread the batter in a spiral motion using the round side of the ladle. Bake until the outer edge of the crepe starts curling up. Flip and bake briefly.
5. If not serving directly, place the crepes on a wire rack until cooled to prevent them from sticking together. The crepes freeze well, but remember to layer them with parchment paper.

Note: Quinoa crepes are protein-rich and gluten-free. To make this recipe even easier, you can use shop-bought pita wraps (but note that most contain gluten).

For the filling
1. Place hummus or avocado slices on half of the wrap. Complete with veggies to taste. Be careful not to overfill!
2. Roll up and secure with 2–3 skewers. Slice it into pieces.

Makes 14–15 crepes.

Easy But Delicious Chili
Recipe by Joanne Kong

Ingredients
- 1/3–1/2 cup onion, chopped
- 1,275 g (3 15-oz cans) of beans (such as kidney, black, great northern), drained and rinsed
- 1 red bell pepper, chopped
- 1/2 cup frozen corn, defrosted
- 800 g (28-oz can) crushed tomatoes
- 2/3 cup cooked farro or other whole-grain
- 1 tsp cumin
- 1 1/2 tsp chili powder

- 1 tsp smoked paprika
- 1/2 tsp garlic powder
- 1 1/2 cups water or vegetable stock
- Optional: chopped cilantro, vegan sour cream

Instructions

1. In a large pot, sauté the onion in a little water until softened.
2. Add the beans, pepper, corn, tomatoes, and whole grains, cooking until well mixed.
3. Add in the spices.
4. Continue simmering for 10–15 minutes, adding vegetable stock or water until desired thickness is reached.
5. Serve along with optional toppings of chives and/or sour cream.

Pasta Carbonara

Recipe by Camila Perussello

Ingredients

- 500 g (18 oz) fusilli pasta
- 180 g (6 oz) smoked tofu
- 1 cup sundried tomatoes
- 1 cup cashew nuts, soaked overnight in cold water (or for 30 minutes in warm water)
- 3 Tbsp nutritional yeast
- Juice of 1–2 limes
- 2–3 cups boiling water
- 1 cup fresh parsley or coriander, chopped
- 1 large onion (white or red)
- 5 garlic cloves
- 2–3 Tbsp olive oil
- Oregano
- Salt and black pepper

Instructions

1. Cook the fusilli pasta according to package directions. While the pasta cooks, prepare the white cream sauce and "bacon."
2. In a pan, sauté the chopped onion and four cloves of chopped garlic with olive oil until golden.
3. Add in the chopped sundried tomatoes. Sauté for a few minutes, then set aside.
4. Drain the soaked cashew nuts and add them to a blender along with the boiling water, lime juice, one raw garlic clove, nutritional yeast, and salt. Blend until smooth and creamy, adjusting salt and lime juice to taste.
5. Drain the cooked pasta and add it to the pan with the sautéed onion, garlic, and sundried tomatoes. Mix in the chopped parsley or coriander and sprinkle with oregano.
6. Pour the white cream sauce over the pasta mixture and stir well to combine.
7. Transfer the creamy pasta carbonara to a serving dish or tray and garnish with additional parsley or coriander leaves.

Makes 4 servings.

Note: The cashew sauce will thicken as it cools down, so make it thinner than you would typically do.

Vegetable & Tempeh Wellington with Shiitake Gravy
Recipe by Marlene Watson-Tara

Ingredients

For the Wellington
- 250 g (9 oz) pack vegan puff pastry
- 225 g (8 oz) pack organic tempeh, cubed and marinated
- 1 bunch spinach, chopped
- 6 medium portobello mushrooms, sliced 1/4-inch thick
- Pinch sea salt
- 2 Tbsp red wine
- 2 garlic cloves, minced
- 2 large leeks (white part only), trimmed and cut into ½-inch slices

- 2 cups celery, thinly sliced
- 2 cups red onion, thinly sliced
- 2 cups carrots, thinly sliced
- 1 Tbsp tamari
- 1/2 tsp dried sage
- 1/2 tsp dried thyme
- 1 large carrot, thinly cut on the diagonal and steamed
- Basil pesto

For braising the tempeh
- 1 Tbsp shoyu
- 1 Tbsp rice mirin
- 1 Tbsp ume plum seasoning
- 1/2 Tbsp freshly squeezed ginger juice
- 1 garlic clove, crushed
- 1/2 tsp dried mixed herbs

For the vegan egg wash
- 1 Tbsp aquafaba (chickpea water)
- 1 Tbsp almond milk
- 1/2 tsp maple syrup or brown rice syrup

Note: It is recommended that the egg wash is prepared before assembling the Wellington.

For the shiitake gravy
- 2 cups button mushrooms, very thinly sliced
- 2 cups fresh shiitake mushrooms, very thinly sliced
- Pinch of sea salt
- 1 Tbsp tamari
- 1 cup rice or almond milk
- 1/2 cup vegetable stock
- 1 tbsp kuzu dissolved in 1/4 cup water

Instructions

For the tempeh
1. Cut the tempeh into bite-sized cubes. Add all the other ingredients to a jar, close the lid tightly, and shake well to mix.
2. Warm a little filtered water in a heavy-based pan over low-medium heat, add the tempeh cubes, and cook covered for 5 minutes.
3. Pour over the marinade, cover, and cook on low heat for 25 minutes, adding water if the pan dries out. Transfer to a large bowl.

For the pastry
1. Follow the instructions on your pastry packet for thawing. Remove the pastry from the box and lay on a baking tray lined with parchment paper. Let it sit for 15 minutes, then gently roll it and let the pastry come to room temperature.

For the greens
1. Bring a small pan of filtered water to a boil. Pop the spinach into a steamer basket. Cover and steam the spinach for 1–2 minutes until wilted. Transfer to a small plate and set aside.

For the mushrooms
1. In a heavy-based pan, heat a little filtered water and cook the mushrooms with a pinch of sea salt for 7–8 minutes.
2. Add the red wine and allow it to soak into the mushrooms; cook until the pan is dry. Remove the mushrooms to a bowl and set aside.

For the filling
1. Using the same pan, add a splash of filtered water and sauté the garlic, leeks, celery, onions, carrots, tamari, and herbs. Cook for 5–7 minutes.
2. Remove from the pan and allow the mixture to cool. Add this mixture to the tempeh bowl, use a paper towel to blot any moisture, then transfer to a dish and chill in the fridge.

Note: The secret to a deliciously juicy yet flaky Wellington is to pat everything dry and ensure it is completely cold before wrapping it in the vegan puff pastry.

For the vegan egg wash
1. Whisk all ingredients together in a bowl.
2. Using a pastry brush, very lightly coat the Wellington. Place the baking tray with the Wellington in the freezer for 10 minutes before repeating with another layer of vegan egg wash. Freeze for a further 10 minutes.

For stuffing the Wellington
1. Preheat the oven to 200°C (392°F), gas 6. Layer the mushrooms onto the prepared pastry sheet, spreading them evenly along the edge of the pastry nearest to you. Layer some filling on top of the mushrooms, then the spinach, and top with a layer of steamed carrots. Add a thin layer of basil pesto along the full length of the filling.
2. Very carefully fold the pastry over the top of the mixture and press down to seal the edges. Trim any excess pastry and crimp around the edges with the back of a fork.
3. Using a sharp knife, score diagonally across the pastry in both directions. Put in a couple of vents by pushing a sharp knife down into the middle of the pastry.
4. Place the baking tray in the oven for 30–35 minutes, or until golden and flaky. Beautifully layered colors of delicious vegetables encased in puff pastry will be the end result, and served with some shiitake gravy is heaven on earth.

For making the shiitake gravy
1. Heat a splash or two of water in a saucepan over medium heat.
2. Add all the mushrooms, sea salt and tamari and sauté for five minutes. Reduce the heat to low and cook, covered, for 10 minutes.
3. Whisk in the milk and stock, then add the kuzu and stir constantly to avoid lumps.
4. Simmer for 15 minutes, or until thickened, whisking often. Add more water if necessary, to reach the desired consistency. Serve as is or blend to a cream.

Makes 8 servings.

Note: Use any remaining filling and leftover pastry to make mini pastries that are great for snacks or picnics. The leftovers also work well as a pie filling.

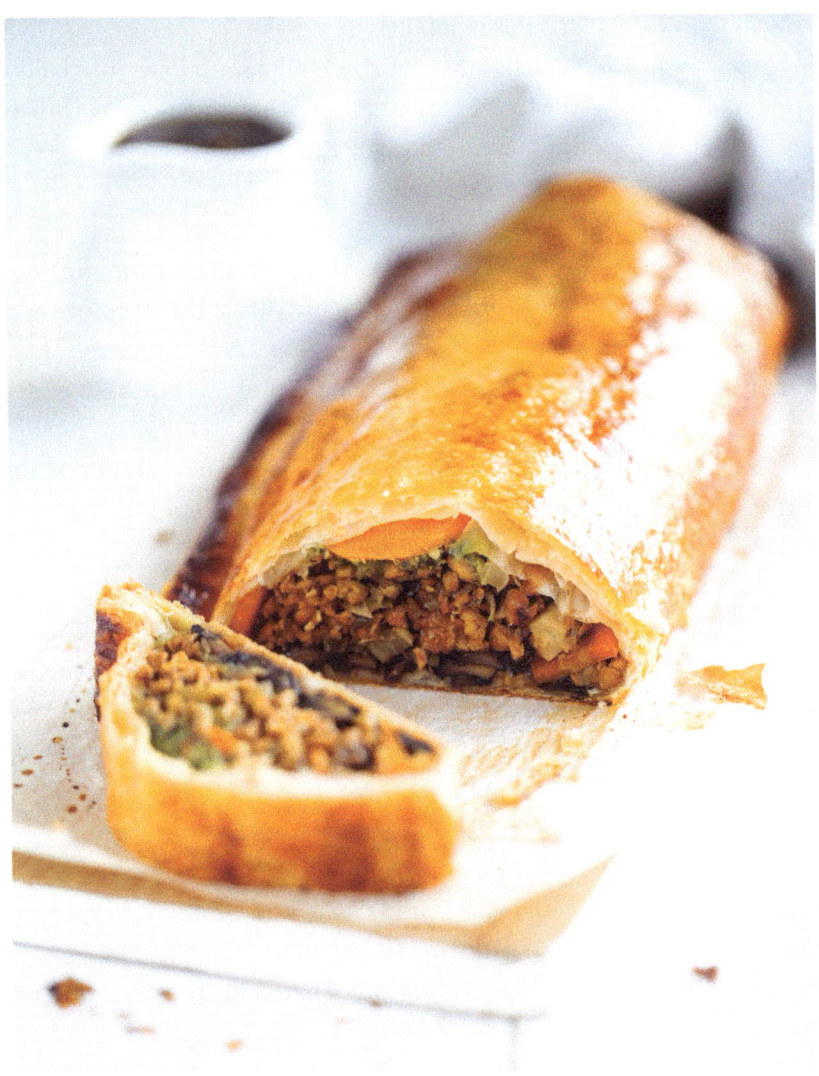

Source: Go Vegan (Lotus Publishing, 2019).

Hearts of Palm Pie

Recipe by Camila Perussello

Ingredients

For the dough
- 1 1/2 cups all-purpose flour
- 1/3 cup olive oil
- 1 Tbsp vegan butter, chilled
- 1/2 cup ice-cold water
- 1/2 teaspoon salt
- Pinch of turmeric
- To glaze: 1 tsp maple syrup mixed with 1 Tbsp water and a pinch of salt

For the filling
- 300 g (10 1/2 oz) hearts of palm
- 220 g (8-oz can) tomato sauce
- 5 ripe tomatoes, diced
- 3 Tbsp concentrated tomato paste (in a tube)
- 3 Tbsp olive oil
- 1 large onion, chopped
- 5 garlic cloves, chopped
- 1 cup leek, chopped
- 1/2 cup green olives
- 1 cup plant-based milk
- 1/2 cup parsley, chopped
- 1 tsp cornstarch dissolved in a little water
- 1 tsp demerara or brown sugar (optional)
- Salt to taste
- Black pepper to taste

Instructions

For the filling
1. In a pan, sauté garlic and onion with olive oil until slightly browned.
2. Add the tomatoes (or tomato sauce) and cook for 2–3 more minutes.
3. Add palms of heart, olives, and tubed tomato paste. Cook for a further 2–3 minutes.
4. Add remaining ingredients and cook for 1–2 minutes. Set aside and let it cool down while you make the dough.

For the dough
1. Sift the flour through a sieve. Add in olive oil, vegan butter, salt, turmeric, and cold water. Adjust quantities of water or flour until you obtain a firm dough that can be rolled out with your fingers.
2. Grease a 24 cm diameter springform pan. Roll out the dough with a rolling pin, lightly flouring the surface to prevent sticking.
3. Cover the bottom and edges of the pan with the dough. Remember to leave some of it to cover the pie (and decorate it, if desired).
4. Add the filling to the pan and cover with dough. You can use molds or stamps to cut the dough and decorate the pie. For instance, overlap stripes and/or arrange cut-out shapes on top of the pie for an artistic effect.
5. Brush the dough with a vegan egg wash (e.g., made of flaxseeds) or a mixture of maple syrup, water, and salt for a glossy finish.

Serves 4.

Note: The sieving step is helpful if you want a flakier and lighter pie crust. For a denser or more rustic texture, you can skip this step and simply mix the flour with the other ingredients. Additionally, cold ingredients are essential to maintain the integrity of the fat in the dough, resulting in a flakier texture during baking.

Refried Bean Tacos with Caramelized Plantains
Recipe by Karoline Mueller

Ingredients
For the tacos
- 8 corn tortillas or tortillas of your choice, warmed or toasted
- 1 small onion, chopped
- 3–4 cloves garlic, chopped, sautéed for 1 minute
- 850 g (2 15-oz cans) of pinto or black beans
- 1/2–1 cup bean liquid or veggie broth
- 1–2 tsp chili powder
- 1 tsp smoked paprika
- 1/2–1 tsp cumin
- 1/2 tsp oregano
- 1/2–1 cup tomatoes, diced, or 85 g (3 oz) tomato paste
- 1–2 Tbsp lime juice
- Salt to taste
- Optional: 1 jalapeño pepper, diced
- Topping options: lettuce, cilantro, fresh tomatoes, avocado, pico de gallo, and salsa

For the plantains
- 3–4 plantains

Note: Buy plantains that are yellow (not green) and ripen until at least half of the skin is black.

Instructions
For the tacos
1. Sauté the onions until golden brown. Use a few tablespoons of water or broth as needed to prevent burning.
2. When the onions are ready, add garlic and optional jalapeño. Sauté for another minute, again adding liquid as needed.

3. Add beans, bean liquid (or veggie broth), and spices. Keep simmering for about 10 minutes to reduce the liquid, stirring regularly.
4. Mash the mixture with a potato masher.
5. Add the tomatoes or tomato paste and heat thoroughly. Finish with lime juice and salt to taste.
6. Fill warmed or toasted tortillas with refried beans, and add any toppings.

For the plantains
1. Peel and cut in half lengthwise.
2. Put the round side down into a pan and heat it at very low heat. Flip after about 10 minutes and cook the flat side until browned. Use a thin-edged spatula to flip. A nonstick pan makes it easier, but a stainless-steel pan works too as long as the heat is kept very low.
3. Bake in the oven at 177°C (350°F) for 30 minutes.

Ramen Bowl with Fresh Daikon & Greens
Recipe by Marlene Tara-Watson

Ingredients
- 250 g (9 oz) organic ramen noodles
- 8 cups filtered water
- 5 garlic cloves, crushed
- 1-inch piece ginger, sliced
- 1 chili, seeded and sliced (optional)
- 1 5-inch piece kombu
- 1 cup spring onions, sliced (reserve some for garnish)
- 3 dried shitake mushrooms
- 1 tsp ground turmeric
- 4 black garlic cloves, sliced
- 1 cup fresh shiitake mushrooms, thinly sliced
- 1/2 Tbsp tamari

- 1/2 Tbsp brown rice vinegar or mirin
- 1 small daikon radish, grated
- Barley or brown rice miso
- 1/4 cup dried wakame seaweed flakes
- 300 g (10 1/2 oz) soft tofu, cubed

Instructions

1. In a medium soup pot, combine water with crushed garlic cloves, ginger, chili, kombu, spring onions, dried shiitake, and turmeric. Leave to soak for at least one hour (preferably overnight to develop a deeper umami flavor).
2. Bring to a boil over medium-high heat. Reduce the heat and simmer partially covered for 30 minutes. Remove from heat, cover, and let it infuse further while cooking the mushrooms.
3. In a large pan, warm a splash of water and sauté the black garlic and mushrooms for 7–8 minutes, until all the liquid released by the mushrooms is evaporated.
4. Add tamari and brown rice vinegar/mirin and cook for another 2 minutes, until all the liquid is absorbed. Remove from the heat and set aside.
5. Strain the broth, pour it back into the pot, and turn the heat to medium-high. Reserve the rehydrated dried shiitake and discard the rest of the solids strained from the broth.
6. Slice the rehydrated shiitake and add back into the broth. When the broth begins to boil, add the noodles and sautéed mushroom mixture to the pot. Cook over low heat for 3–5 minutes, until the noodles are soft but not mushy.
7. In a small bowl, combine the miso paste with half a cup of the broth until smooth.
8. Use approximately one teaspoon of miso per cup of soup. Add the miso to the soup pot and mix to incorporate.
9. Stir in the wakame seaweed, if using. Taste broth for salt and add a splash of tamari if more salt is needed.
10. Serve right away garnished with sliced spring onion, cubed tofu, grated daikon, and toasted sesame seeds. Store the leftovers in the refrigerator for up to 3 days.

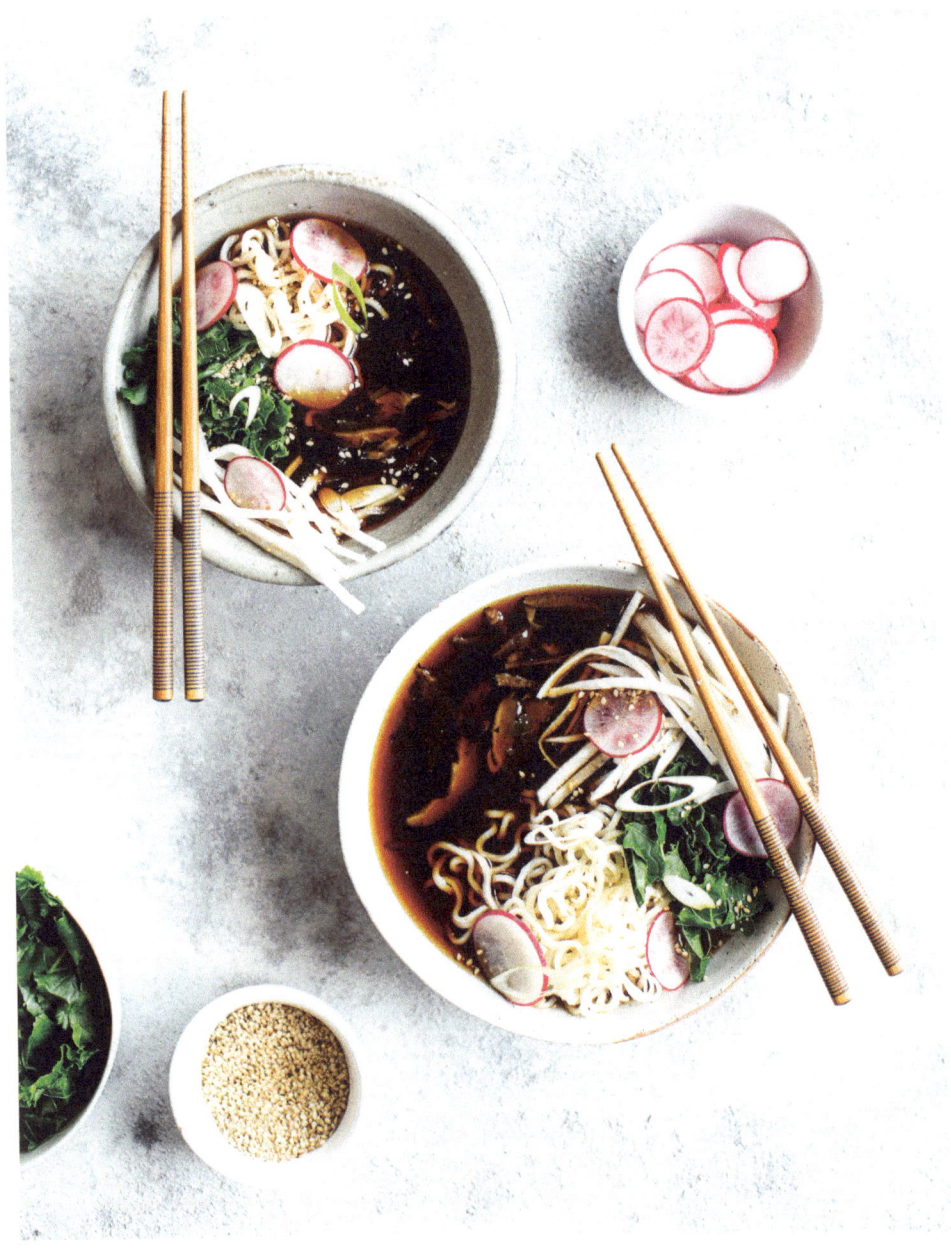

Source: Go Vegan (Lotus Publishing, 2019).

Instant Pot-Atouille
Recipe by Chef AJ

Ingredients
- 1/2 cup water
- 230 g (8 oz) yellow Crookneck squash
- 230 g (8 oz) green zucchini
- 340 g (12 oz) Chinese or Japanese Eggplant
- 1 orange bell pepper (about 230 g)
- 2–3 portobello mushrooms (about 170 g)
- 1/2 red onion, chopped (about 170 g)
- 680 g (1.5 pounds) Yukon Gold potatoes
- 820 g (2 14.5-oz cans) Muir Glen Salt-Free Fire Roasted Tomatoes
- 1/2 cup fresh basil, finely chopped into threads (chiffonade cut)

Instructions
1. Place all ingredients, except for the fresh basil, in an 8-quart Instant Pot electric pressure cooker and cook on high pressure for 10 minutes.
2. Release pressure and stir in the basil.
3. Serve with rice if desired (I like to add 2–3 cups of cooked rice to the stew before serving). Sprinkle *Enlightened Faux Parmesan* (see recipe on p. 127 of my book *The Secrets to Ultimate Weight Loss*)

Note: If you don't have the 8-quart Instant Pot, cut the recipe in half. Because I like starch with my starch, I still enjoy serving it with brown rice to soak up some of the juice.

Linguine with Artichoke Hearts
Recipe by Nancy Arenas

Ingredients
- 340 g (12 oz) linguine pasta
- 425 g (15 oz) artichoke hearts, quartered
- 1 cup textured vegetable protein (TVP)
- 1/2–1 cup marinara sauce
- Vegan cheese (you can use shredded cheese, or tear up cheese slices to melt easier)
- Italian seasoning
- Basil
- Oregano
- Garlic powder
- 1 Tbsp nutritional yeast

Instructions
1. Cook the pasta according to package directions. Drain the cooked pasta.
2. In a large skillet, add the artichoke hearts, marinara sauce, and TVP.
3. Season to taste with Italian seasoning, basil, oregano, and garlic powder. Mix in the nutritional yeast.
4. Add the vegan cheese and cook for 10 minutes.
5. Add the cooked pasta to the skillet, gently fold it in, and cook for 5 minutes.

Feijoada (Brazilian Bean Stew)
Recipe by Camila Perussello

Ingredients
- 500 g (17 1/2 oz) black beans (dried)
- 500 mL (2 cups) water (or enough to cover the beans in the cooking pan)
- 400 g (14 oz) smoked tofu, cubed
- 3–4 vegan sausages, thickly sliced
- 100 mL (1/2 cup) soy sauce

- 200 g (7 oz) mushrooms
- 2 onions
- 7 garlic cloves
- 1/2 cup green onions, chopped
- 3 Tbsp olive oil
- 3 bay leaves
- Salt to taste
- Black pepper to taste
- Optional: 1 Tbsp liquid smoke or 100 mL of lapsang souchong tea for a stronger smoky flavor

Instructions

1. Soak the black beans in water for at least 8 hours. This process helps release phytates, reducing bloating for those sensitive to beans and other legumes. As a bonus, the beans will cook faster, and their nutrients will be better preserved.
2. Drain the beans, add them to a pan or pressure cooker, and cover with water. Add salt and bay leaves. Cook until tender (around 12–15 minutes in the pressure cooker).
3. While the beans are cooking, dice the tofu block into small cubes and slice the sausages. Put them into a bowl with soy sauce and marinate for around 10 minutes.
4. Remove excess soy sauce from the tofu and sausage and grill them until golden on all sides. Use a little olive oil to grease the pan if needed. Set aside.
5. In another pan, sauté onions and garlic in olive oil until golden. Set aside.
6. Once the beans are soft enough to be pierced with a fork (but not sloshy!), mix beans, sausages, tofu, mushrooms, pepper, and the sautéed onions and garlic. If desired, add the liquid smoke or tea at this point. Simmer for another 5–10 minutes, without a lid. You want a rich and thick stew. If the stew is too thin, continue simmering to allow excess liquid to evaporate and the stew to thicken naturally. You can also use a spoon or a potato masher to lightly mash some of the beans against the side of the pot. This helps thicken the stew. Alternatively, add a small amount of cornstarch mixed with water to thicken the stew.

7. When the desired thickness is reached, add in spring onions, mix, and adjust the salt and pepper to taste. Serve while hot.

Note: Traditionally, feijoada is served with fluffy white or brown rice, lightly sautéed collard greens (*couve à mineira*), and a crunchy side dish called *farofa*. The many variations of farofa include cassava flour, ripe bananas, and sautéed onions. The meal is typically garnished with orange slices to add color and a refreshing citrusy flavor that cuts through the richness of the feijoada.

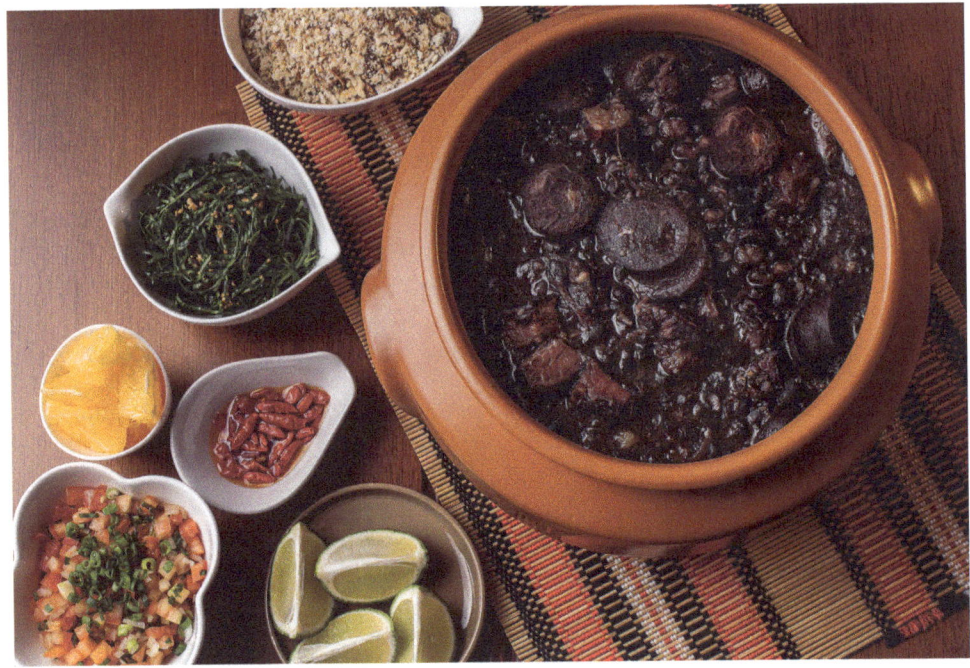

Photo credit: Flavia Novais (www.istockphoto.com).

Portobello Mushroom Stroganoff

Recipe by Marlene Watson-Tara

Ingredients

For the sauce

- 1 cup cashews, soaked overnight
- 1 1/2 cups filtered water
- 1 Tbsp ume plum vinegar
- 1 heaped Tbsp tahini
- 1 Tbsp tamari or shoyu

For the stroganoff

- 3 cups portobello mushrooms, very thinly sliced
- 1 large onion, thinly sliced
- 1 shallot, thinly sliced
- 2 cloves garlic, minced
- 1 umami instant stock sachet dissolved in 2 cups warm filtered water
- 1 1/2 tsp Seaweed Agogo Italian Herb Mix
- 1/2 cup tightly packed fresh parsley, chopped

For garnishing

- Black sesame seeds
- Chopped coriander
- Lemon zest

Instructions

1. Warm a splash or two of filtered water in a heavy-based pot on a medium-low flame. Sauté the mushrooms, onion, shallot, and garlic for 5 minutes.
2. Reduce the heat to low and add the umami stock and the Seaweed Agogo Italian Herb Mix. Cover and simmer for 15 minutes.
3. Drain the cashews from their soaking water and place them in a blender with the remaining sauce ingredients. Blend to a cream.
4. Add the cashew cream to the pot mixture, stirring well to combine. Cook, covered, on a low simmer for 15 minutes. Add water to reach the desired consistency. The stroganoff will thicken as it sits, so make sure to thin slightly before serving.
5. Stir in the chopped parsley. Serve in bowls, garnished with black sesame seeds, chopped coriander, and lemon zest. Delicious served on a bed of fluffy basmati rice.

Makes 4–6 servings.

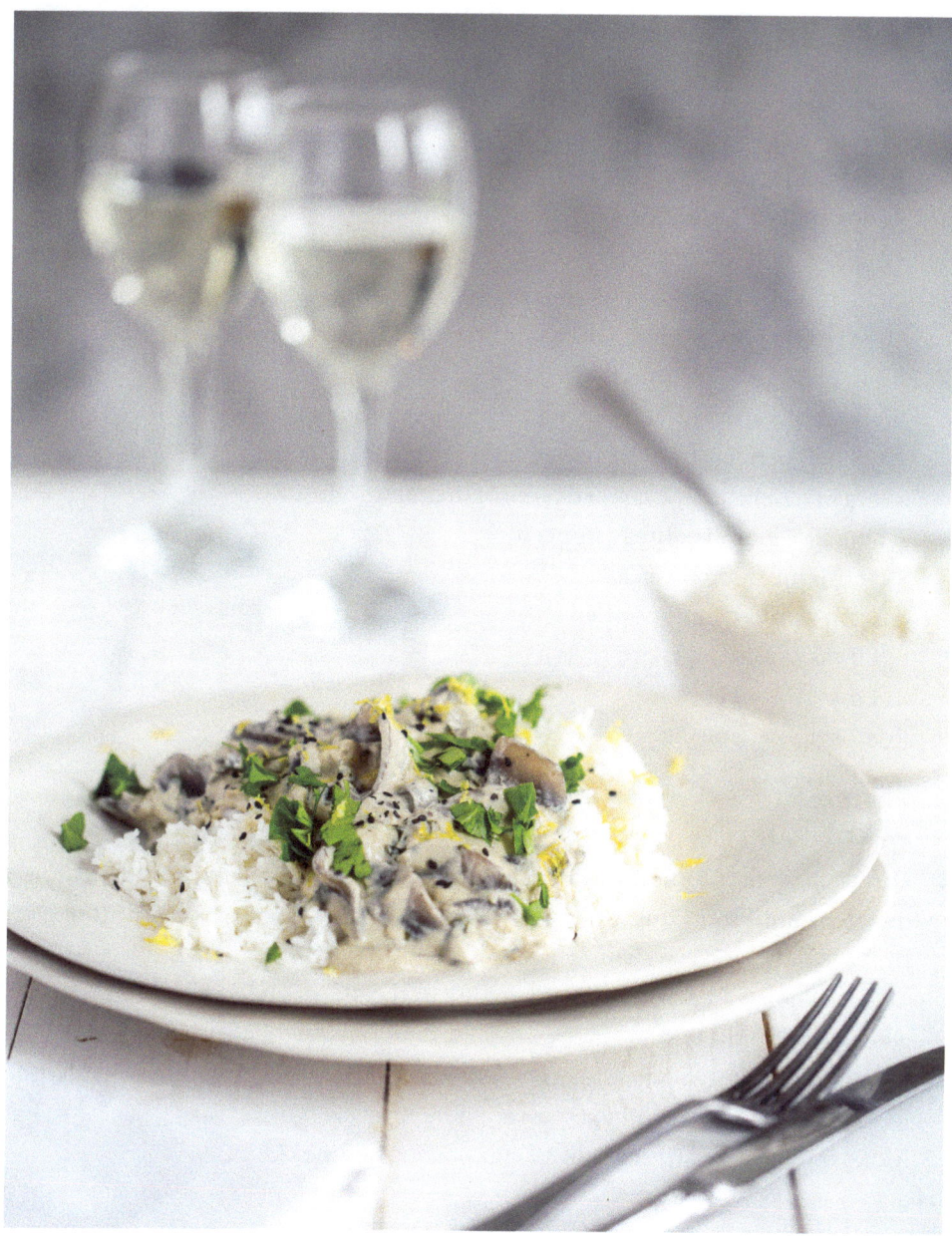

Source: Go Vegan (Lotus Publishing, 2019).

Chipotle Bean Burgers
Recipe by Chef AJ

Ingredients
- 4 15-oz cans salt-free black beans, rinsed and drained (or 6 cups cooked beans)
- 4 cups cooked brown rice
- 4 cups cooked and mashed sweet potato (I prefer to use the starchier Hannah Yams rather than mushy orange ones)
- 410 g (14.5-oz can) Muir Glen Salt-Free Fire Roasted Tomatoes
- 1 cup red onion, chopped
- 8 cloves of garlic, minced or put through a garlic press
- 1 red bell pepper, finely chopped (approximately 1 cup)
- 1 large carrot, finely chopped (approximately 1 cup)
- 1 bunch of cilantro, finely minced
- 12 Tbsp nutritional yeast
- 4 Tbsp salt-free chili powder
- 1 Tbsp smoked paprika
- 1 Tbsp ground cumin
- 1 tsp chipotle powder

Instructions
1. Preheat the oven to 204°C (400°F).
2. Drain the can of tomatoes and sauté the onion in the liquid from the canned tomatoes until soft. You can puree the tomatoes in a food processor fitted with the "S" blade or leave them whole.
3. Add the chopped carrot, bell pepper, and garlic, and sauté until soft and cooked (about 10–15 minutes).
4. Combine all ingredients in a large bowl and stir to mix. I prefer to use latex-free food service gloves. Chill for several hours or overnight.
5. Make individual patties out of ½ cup portions of the mixture.

6. Place patties on the baking sheet and bake for 30–45 minutes until you can flip them over easily without sticking. After you flip them, bake for another 20–30 minutes.

Makes 24 burgers. These freeze very well.

Note: Everyone who tastes these, even hard-core carnivores, says these are the best bean burgers they have ever tasted! Serve these flavorful, filling burgers with all the fixings, such as sliced tomatoes, onions, and salt-free condiments, and use large butter lettuce leaves or potato waffles as buns. They can also be crumbled and served over a salad or used as a delicious filling for a baked potato. You can watch me make these on *Healthy Living with Chef AJ* here: https://www.youtube.com/watch?v=AewkOvhDWuY&t=301s.

6.3 Sauces & Sides

Tortilla Chips
Recipe by Karoline Mueller

Ingredients
- 2–3 corn tortillas per person

Instructions
1. Cut tortillas into quarters. Sprinkle with lime juice and salt to taste.
2. Toast about 10–15 minutes until crisp, in a toaster oven, air fryer, or bake at 204°C (400°F) in a conventional oven. If using the oven, a pizza stone is useful but not necessary.

Mango Salsa
Recipe by Jim McGehee

Ingredients
- 1 large mango, 2 small ones, or around 140 g frozen mangos, diced (other fruits like pineapple or peaches work well too)
- 1 large tomato or a handful of cherry tomatoes, diced
- 1 Tbsp jalapeño, finely diced, or ½ tsp crushed red pepper
- 3 Tbsp lime juice
- 1/4 cup cilantro, minced

Instructions
1. Mix all ingredients and enjoy! Goes really well with the tortilla chips above.

Algarvian Guacamole
Recipe by Camila Perussello

Ingredients
- 1 medium ripe avocado, diced
- 1 ripe tomato, diced
- 1/2 cup red onion, thinly chopped
- Juice of one lime
- 1 tsp olive oil
- 1 tsp garlic powder
- 1/4 cup cilantro, chopped
- 1 Tbsp black sesame seeds, for topping
- Salt, if necessary

Instructions
1. Mix all ingredients (except for the sesame) and adjust the flavor to your preference with more lime juice, olive oil, or salt.
2. Add sesame seeds on top and serve it.

Note: This guacamole version pairs perfectly with tortilla chips, crackers, and sourdough bread. It is also fantastic on avocado toast!

Asparagus with Vegan Hollandaise Sauce
Recipe by Marlene Watson-Tara

Ingredients
- 1 large bunch asparagus, trimmed
- 1 Tbsp fresh lemon juice
- 1 tsp tamari or shoyu
- 2 Tbsp nutritional yeast
- 1 tsp Dijon mustard
- 1/2 tsp tahini
- 1/2 cup soft silken tofu, drained
- 1/4 tsp turmeric
- Sprinkling of turmeric to garnish

Instructions

1. Bring a small pot of filtered water to a boil. Pop the asparagus into a steamer basket. Cover and steam the asparagus for 4–6 minutes or just until crisp and tender.
2. Meanwhile, blend all the other ingredients into a smooth cream in a high-speed blender.
3. Transfer to a small saucepan and cook over low heat, stirring constantly until heated through.
4. Arrange the hot asparagus on a serving platter and pour the sauce over top. Serve immediately and dust lightly with turmeric.

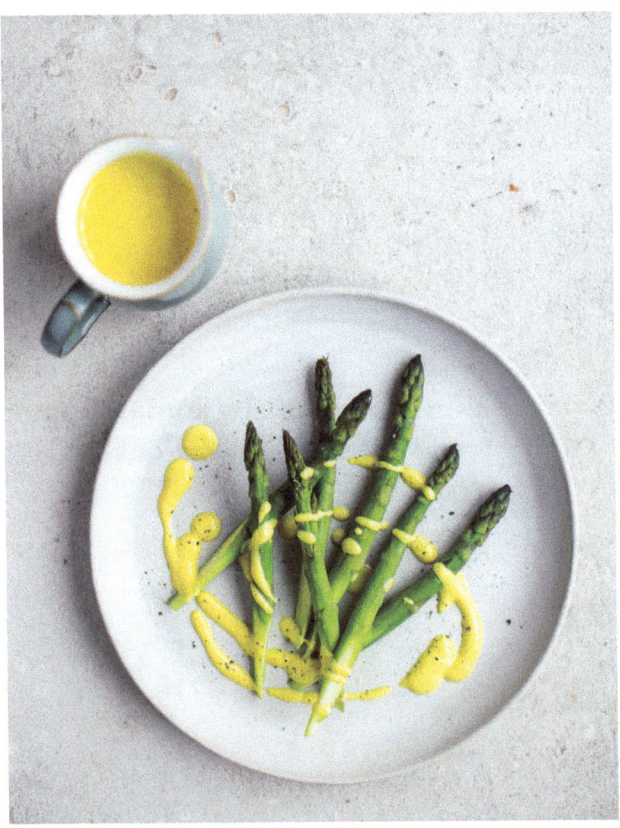

Source: Go Vegan (Lotus Publishing, 2019).

Homemade Cucumber Pickles
Recipe by Jim McGehee

Ingredients
- 1 package Persian cucumbers (about 6) or 1 English cucumber, sliced
- 1 onion, finely sliced
- 1 tsp yellow mustard seeds
- 1 cup rice vinegar
- 2 cups water
- Optional: 1/2 tsp sugar, spices, and herbs (e.g., dill and thyme)

Instructions
1. Layer cucumber and onion slices in a sealable dish.
2. Sprinkle with mustard seeds and optional spices.
3. Mix vinegar and water in a 1:2 ratio.
4. Cover vegetables well with liquid and marinate in the refrigerator. They will keep for several weeks.

Simple Marinara Sauce
Recipe by Karoline Mueller

Ingredients
- 425 g (15 oz) canned tomatoes
- 85–115 g (3–4 oz) tomato paste
- 2 tsp onion powder
- 2 tsp garlic powder
- 1/2 tsp black pepper
- 2 tsp Italian herb blend, or mix 1/2 tsp thyme, 1/2 tsp oregano, and 1 tsp basil

Instructions
1. Blend all ingredients and heat up.

6.4 Soups & Breads

Kale & Quinoa Soup
Recipe by Nancy Arenas

Ingredients
- 2 1/2 quarts of water
- 1 bunch of kale
- 2 cups quinoa
- Adobo seasoning
- Garlic
- Onion powder
- Turmeric
- Oregano
- Cilantro
- Cumin
- Salt
- 2 vegan bouillon cubes
- 2 packets of Sazón seasoning

Instructions
1. In a pot, combine water, quinoa, and kale.
2. Add two vegan bouillon cubes and season with spices and salt to taste.
3. Mix in the Sazón seasoning and cook until the quinoa and kale have softened. Adjust the seasonings according to your taste preferences.

Spicy Brown Lentil Soup with Sour Cream

Recipe by Marlene Watson-Tara

Ingredients

- 1 1/2 cups brown lentils (rinsed and soaked for 30 minutes)
- 2 Tbsp vegetable stock or filtered water
- 2 shallots, finely chopped
- 1 leek, very finely sliced
- 1 small squash, cut into small cubes
- 1 courgette, cut into small cubes
- 1 sweet potato, peeled and cut into small cubes
- 1 parsnip, peeled and cut into small cubes
- 1 cup fresh or frozen sweetcorn
- Pinch sea salt
- 2 tsp dried basil
- 1 tsp ground cumin
- 1 Tbsp ground coriander
- 1/2 tsp chili powder (optional)
- 2 umami instant stock sachets dissolved in 6 cups filtered water
- Shoyu to taste
- Vegan sour cream
- Chopped parsley or coriander

Instructions

1. Heat the water or stock in a large pot and cook the shallots and leek over a low heat for 5–7 minutes.
2. Add the squash, courgette, sweet potato, parsnip, sweetcorn, salt, basil, and spices. Cook for 5 minutes.
3. Pour in the stock, cover, and bring to a boil.
4. Add the lentils and cook on low heat, covered, for 20–25 minutes, until the soup starts to thicken. Add more water to reach the desired consistency.
5. Using a stick blender, half-purée the soup so it is thick and creamy but not completely smooth. Adjust the seasoning with shoyu or tamari if desired. Serve in warmed bowls topped with some sour cream. Garnish with chopped parsley or coriander and serve with warmed naan bread.

Makes 6–8 servings.

Note: This soup is a classic recipe that can be made with pretty much any legume. Despite color changes, red lentils, yellow lentils, chickpeas, and beans will all work great with this recipe.

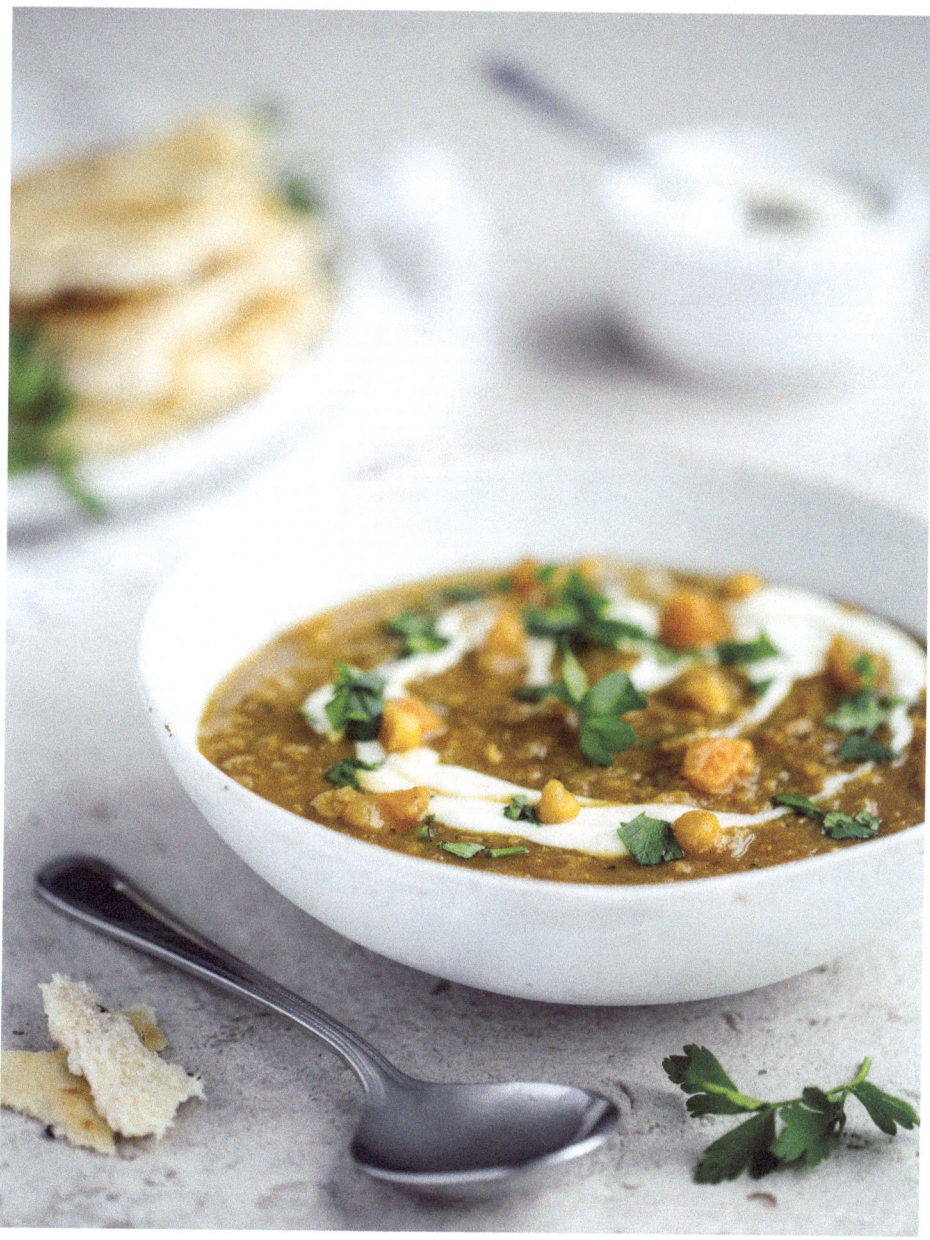

Source: Go Vegan (Lotus Publishing, 2019).

Focaccia al Rosmarino
Recipe by Camila Perussello

Ingredients
- 500 g (17 1/2 oz) wheat flour
- 10 g (.35 oz) dried yeast
- 250–300 mL (1–1 1/3 c) water, lukewarm
- 30 mL (6 tsp) extra virgin olive oil
- Rosemary leaves, preferably fresh (for the surface)
- Table salt (for the dough)
- Coarse salt (for the surface)
- Extra virgin olive oil (for the surface)
- Optional: 1 Tbsp sugar to boost yeast activity and produce a softer, more aromatic dough.

Instructions
1. In a cup, pour some of the lukewarm water and add the dry yeast and sugar. Stir well with a spoon to dissolve the solids, and let it sit for about 10 minutes. By this time, you will have a nice fluffy foam, meaning the microorganisms are active.
2. In a large bowl, add flour, olive oil, the mixture above, salt, and the remaining water. Knead for a few minutes with your fingers until you get a soft, homogeneous dough. Adjust with more water or flour if necessary.
3. Cover the focaccia dough bowl with plastic wrap and place it somewhere warm and draft-free (e.g., in a cabinet or turned-off oven). Allow it to rise for 2 hours or until it doubles in volume.
4. After the rising time, transfer the dough to a well-oiled or silicone baking tray. Using your fingertips, gently spread the dough out to cover the tray evenly.
5. Sprinkle the surface of the focaccia with extra virgin olive oil, coarse salt, and fresh rosemary.
6. Let it rise for another hour, covered with a clean cloth.
7. Bake in a preheated oven at 200°C (392°F) for 20–25 minutes or until slightly golden on the surface.

Creamy Mushroom Soup with Savory Cashew Cream

Recipe by Marlene Watson-Tara

Ingredients

For the cashew cream

- 1/2 cup cashews, soaked overnight
- 1/4 cup filtered water
- 1 tsp fresh lemon juice
- 1 tsp ume plum seasoning

For the soup

- 4 large dried shiitake mushrooms
- 1 cup dried maitake mushrooms, tightly packed
- 2 cups fresh mushrooms, such as shiitake and white button, chopped
- 2 cups spring onions, finely chopped
- Ground black pepper (optional) to taste
- 1/2 tsp dried dill
- 2 cloves garlic, minced
- 1 Tbsp freshly squeezed lemon juice
- 2 Tbsp rice mirin
- 1 umami instant stock sachet dissolved in 1/2 cup warm filtered water
- 2 Tbsp all-purpose flour
- 1/2 cup savory cashew cream, plus a little more for garnish
- 2 Tbsp chives, minced

Instructions

For the cashew cream
1. Place cashews in a bowl, cover with filtered water, and soak overnight.
2. Rinse and place the drained cashews in a high-speed blender. Add the remaining ingredients. Blend on high until super-smooth. You might have to stop to scrape down the blender now and then or add a touch more water. Thin to your desired consistency. Transfer into a small airtight container and chill in the fridge to thicken.

For the soup
1. Soak the dried mushrooms in 4 cups of lukewarm filtered water for one hour. Drain and reserve the soaking water to use as part of the stock. This will give the soup a delicious umami taste.
2. Slice the mushrooms, discarding the stems from the dried shiitakes. Warm a splash or two of water in a heavy-based pot. Add the mushrooms, spring onions, pepper, dill, garlic, and lemon juice. Cook for 2 minutes, stirring frequently.
3. Increase the heat slightly and add the rice mirin. Simmer for 3 minutes or until the liquid is reduced slightly. Whisk the flour into the mixture along with a splash or two of water, stirring well to avoid lumps.
4. Add the stock and soaking liquid from the dried mushrooms. Bring to a boil and reduce the heat to medium-low. Cover and simmer for 30 minutes. Transfer to a blender and purée until smooth.
5. Return to the pot and add the cashew cream. Add extra water to achieve your desired consistency. Serve in warm bowls and add the minced chives and two or three swirls of the cream.

Makes 4–6 servings.

Note: The secret to this rich soup is to use a combination of dried and fresh mushrooms. This will give the soup a much richer color and flavor. You only require a small portion to feel satisfied by the deep, earthy flavors.

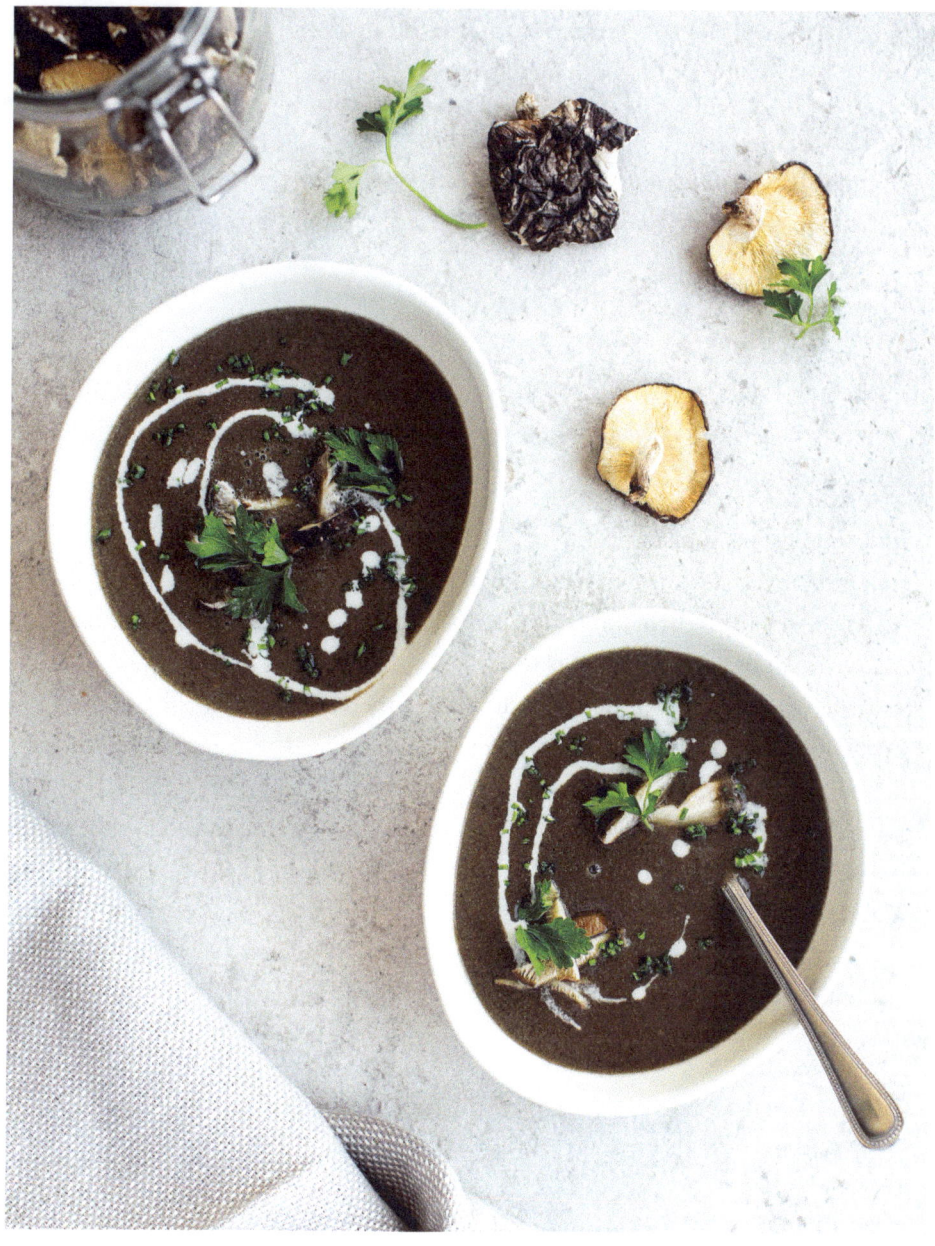

Source: Go Vegan (Lotus Publishing, 2019).

Yummy Spelt Bread

Recipe by Christoph Wagner

Ingredients
- 2 cups lukewarm water
- 1 1/2 tsp active dry yeast
- 2 1/2 cups spelt flour
- 1/2 cup ground flaxseeds
- 1/2 tsp salt
- 1–2 cups of nuts, seeds, and/or dried fruits (raisins, walnuts, pecans, sunflower seeds, whole flaxseeds, chia seeds—whatever you have in the pantry!)

Instructions
1. In a small bowl, whisk together the water and yeast and let sit for 10 minutes.
2. In a large bowl, mix the dry ingredients.
3. Add the wet ingredients and mix with a spoon. The dough should be sticky. Add 1 or 2 Tbsp of water if it is too thick.
4. Transfer the dough to a loaf pan (use parchment paper or a silicone loaf pan). Let sit for about 1 hour for the dough to rest and rise. Preheat the oven to 177°C (350°F).
5. Bake the bread for around 45 minutes. When done, the bread should be brown on top, and when checking with a thin fork or baking needle, it should come out clean.

6.5 Salads & Sandwiches

Watermelon Salad
Recipe by Nancy Arenas

Ingredients
- Watermelon
- Cucumber
- Mint
- Lime juice
- Tajin (Mexican spice blend)
- Chili powder

Instructions
1. Cut the watermelon and cucumber into cubes.
2. In a mixing bowl, combine the watermelon and cucumber, and add mint, lime juice, Tajin, and chili powder to taste. Mix well.

Mediterranean Chickpea Salad Sandwich
Recipe by Marlene Tara-Watson

Ingredients
- Sprouted bread
- 1 cup hummus
- 3 cups cooked chickpeas
- 1 small red onion, shaved
- 1/2 cup artichoke hearts, thinly sliced
- 1/2 cup Kalamata olives, halved
- 1 tsp dried dill
- 1 tsp garlic flakes
- Juice of 1/2 lemon
- Watercress

Instructions

1. In a large mixing bowl, add the chickpeas to the hummus. Using the back of a fork or a potato masher, roughly mash about 3/4 of the chickpeas, leaving some whole.
2. Add in the remaining ingredients and mix well to combine. Serve chilled or at room temperature. Store leftovers in the refrigerator for up to a week in an airtight container. Use this chickpea mixture in lettuce wraps, on a bed of leafy greens with sliced cucumbers and tomatoes, or scoop up with crackers or vegetable crudités. You can also top with some pickled red onions and mashed avocado.

Note: Sprouted bread is made from whole grains that have been allowed to sprout, that is, to germinate, before being milled into flour. There are a few different types of sprouted grain bread. Some are made with added flour, some with added gluten, and others (such as Essene bread) are made with very few additional ingredients.

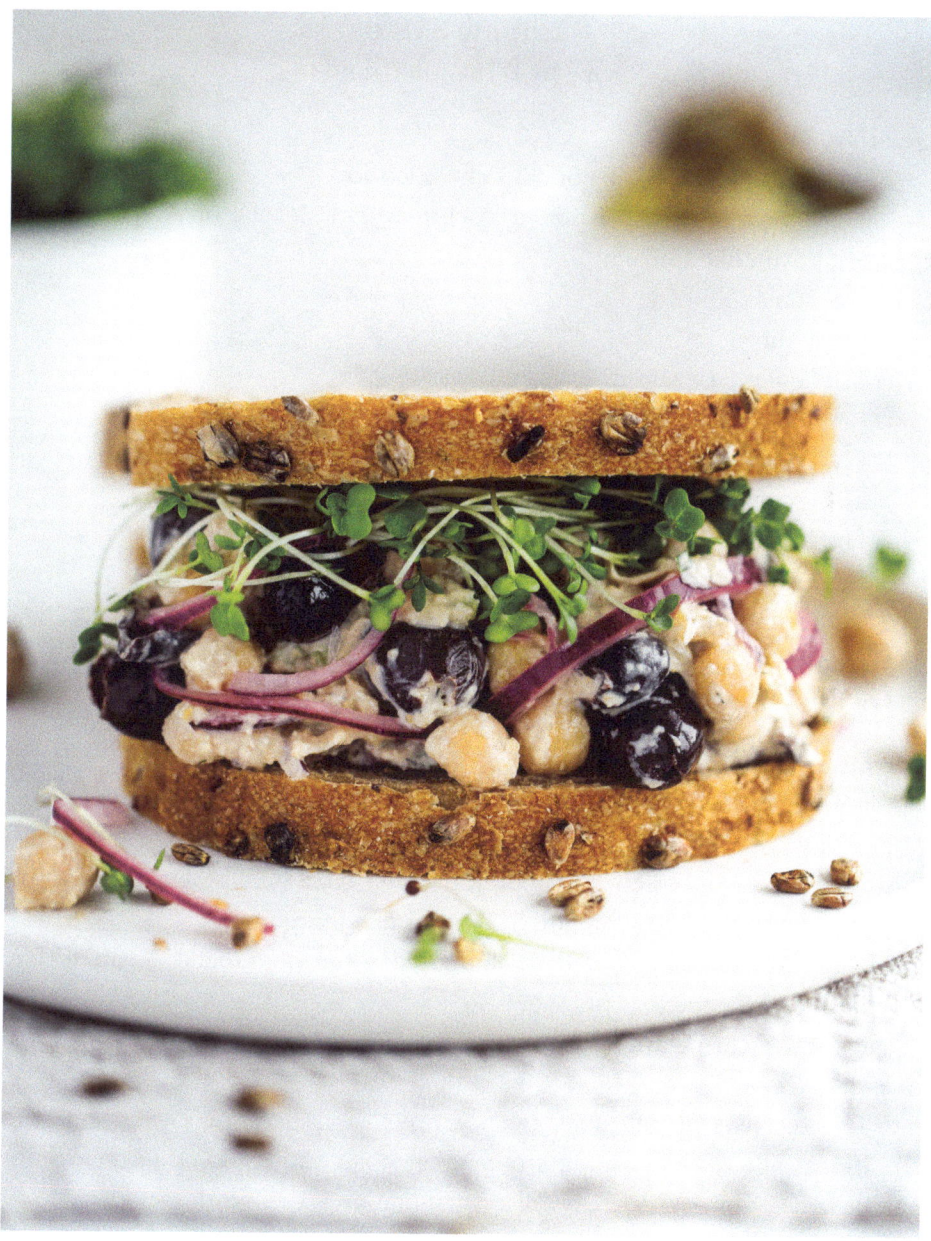

Source: Go Vegan (Lotus Publishing, 2019).

Rainbow Salad
Recipe by Fernando Grando

Ingredients
- 200 g (approximately 1/2 pound) iceberg lettuce
- 100 g (approximately 1/4 pound) rocket/arugula leaves (or alternative dark green leaves, like spinach)
- 1 large tomato, diced
- 1 carrot, diced
- 1/2 stalk of celery, sliced
- 1/4 red onion, diced
- 1/4 bell pepper (color of preference), diced
- 7 large green olives, diced
- 2 Tbsp sweetcorn
- 3 Tbsp extra virgin olive oil (or add to taste)
- 2 Tbsp white wine vinegar or juice of ½ lime
- Garlic powder, to taste
- Oregano, to taste

Instructions
1. In a large bowl, mix the lettuce and rocket. You may choose to slice them a little more if you prefer smaller leaves.
2. Add the onions, mix well, and pour in the olive oil. This way, leaves and onions absorb the oil while you prepare the remaining ingredients.
3. Add in carrots, pepper, and tomatoes. Mix the ingredients again to have uniformly distributed colors.
4. Olives, sweetcorn, garlic powder, and oregano go last.

Serves 2.

Note: This recipe is very flexible, and you are encouraged to try variations, such as replacing ingredients or adding other vegetables and legumes (e.g., cucumber, beetroot, green beans, chickpeas). Your imagination is the limit!

Crunchy Tempeh Salad
Recipe by Nancy Arenas

Ingredients
- 230 g (1 8-oz package) tempeh
- 1/2 stalk of celery
- 3 Tbsp of red onion, finely chopped
- 2 Tbsp of tamari
- 1/2 tsp of liquid smoke
- Walnuts or almonds
- Garlic
- Salt
- Oregano
- Turmeric
- Cilantro
- 1 tsp of sesame seed oil
- Vegan mayonnaise (to taste)

Instructions
1. Break up the tempeh in a bowl. Add celery and onion, and mix well.
2. Add the remaining dry ingredients.
3. Mix in the sesame seed oil, liquid smoke, and tamari. Continue mixing.
4. Add vegan mayo to achieve your desired consistency and mix thoroughly.

Chickpea & Artichoke Salad
Recipe by Nancy Poznak

Ingredients
- 1,250 g (44-oz can) chickpeas, drained and rinsed
- 396 g (14-oz can) artichoke hearts, drained well and chopped into small pieces
- 1/2 cup hemp hearts
- 3 Tbsp vinaigrette dressing (I use Briana's Organic French Vinaigrette)
- 1/4 cup red onion, chopped fine

- 3 Tbsp mustard seed powder
- 1/4 tsp black pepper
- 1/4 tsp salt
- 2 Tbsp garlic powder (not granulated and not garlic salt)
- Tahini or vegan mayonnaise
- Optional: Veggies that have density and will not add moisture, such as carrots and celery

Instructions

1. Mix everything well, then add some tahini or vegan mayo according to your taste.
2. Mix well. It is best to use a mixer to blend, at low speed. Be careful not to overmix.

Crispy Sweet & Sour Tempeh Sourdough Sandwich

Recipe by Marlene Watson-Tara

Ingredients

For the tempeh
- 200 g (7 oz) tempeh sliced into thin strips
- 3 Tbsp balsamic vinegar
- 2 Tbsp maple syrup
- 1 Tbsp tamari
- 1 garlic clove, crushed
- 1/2 tsp paprika

- Bread or bun, toasted
- Vegan mayonnaise
- Red onion, slivers
- Lettuce leaves
- Ketchup
- Sauerkraut
- Sprouts of choice

Instructions

1. Place the tempeh strips in a single layer into a shallow dish.
2. In a small bowl, whisk together the vinegar, maple syrup, tamari, garlic, and paprika. Pour over the tempeh to cover and let marinate for one hour, flipping the tempeh once or twice.
3. Preheat the grill to 200°C (392°F). Remove the tempeh from the marinade and place it on the grill. Cook until golden and crispy, about 7–8 minutes per side.
4. Toast the bread. Spread one half of the bread with a generous portion of mayonnaise and add some red onion. Place cooked tempeh slices on top, followed by lettuce leaves, and top with some ketchup, sauerkraut, and sprouts. Serve immediately.

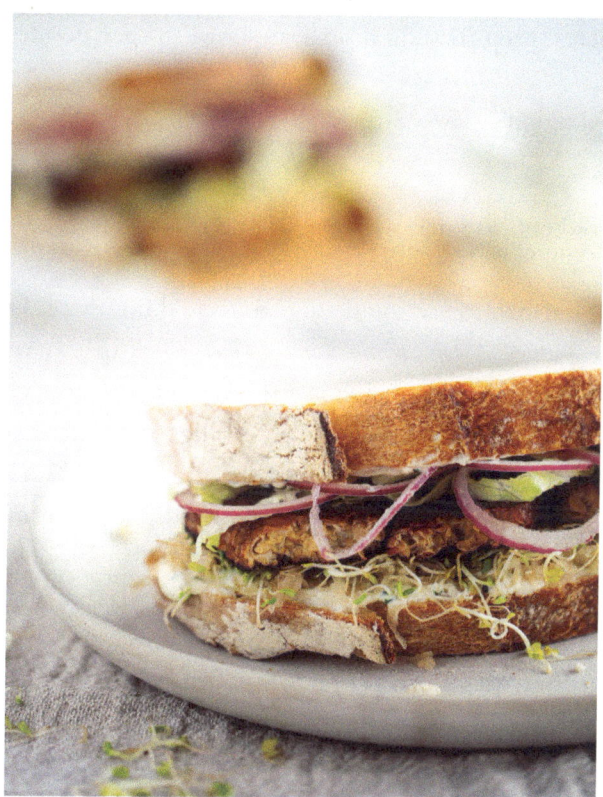

Source: Go Vegan (Lotus Publishing, 2019).

Chef AJ's House Salad

Ingredients

- 3 heads of Romaine lettuce, chopped finely
- 450 g (1 pound) Persian cucumbers, finely chopped
- 450 g (1 pound) bag riced broccoli or riced cauliflower
- 225 g (1/2 pound) shredded carrots
- 225 g (1/2 pound) shredded purple carrots
- 450 g (1 pound) purple grapes, sliced in half
- 1 cup fresh mint, chopped finely
- 4 cups (or more) cooked wild rice
- Shredded beets (keep these in a separate bowl so they do not turn the entire salad pink)
- Chopped red onion

Instructions

1. Chop all ingredients as finely as possible, and that's all!

Note 1: If you would like to see me demonstrate making this salad, please check out my YouTube video, *A Day in the Life of Chef AJ:* https://www.youtube.com/watch?v=3mADxtiCCX8. This recipe is just a template to give you ideas on how to create amazing salads. Obviously, only put in ingredients that you like and will actually eat! Feel free to vary or substitute the grain, or add a different starch like beans, corn, or cooked sweet potato. You can also use alternative herbs, like fresh basil, cilantro, or Italian parsley. If grapes are not in season, try fresh apples, grapefruit, oranges, pears, or pomegranate seeds. With fresh fruit in a salad, salad dressing becomes optional. I recommend including starch in your salad (or eating it immediately afterwards) for satiety.

Note 2: For the best salad-eating experience possible, try to incorporate all the components of my *Secrets to Superior Salad Satisfaction*:

Salad: Romaine or other lettuce

Salty: Finely chopped greens like kale, chard, celery, or some dulse

Sauce: *Barefoot Dressing* (https://www.youtube.com/watch?v=Tltf-qRmFG4) or *House Dressing* 2.0 (https://www.youtube.com/watch?v=2ErHKczzMR8) or your favorite SOS (salt, oil, sugar)-free dressing

Savory: Arugula, onion

Snap: Something crunchy like celery, jicama, or water chestnuts

Sour: A lime or lemon juice squeezed over the salad or vinegar

Specialty: Add optional leftovers such as *Balsamic Dijon Glazed Brussels Sprouts* (see recipe on p. 123 of my book *The Secrets to Ultimate Weight Loss*)

Starchy: Wild rice or other cooked grain like brown rice, millet, or quinoa, or any cooked legume, potato, sweet potato, or squash. Cooked cubes of butternut or kabocha squash are great!

Sweet: Grapes or other fruit

6.6 Desserts

Irresistible Chocolate Mousse
Recipe by Christoph Wagner

Ingredients

400 g (14 oz) silken tofu (super soft)

200 g (7 oz) vegan dark chocolate, approximately 60% cacao content

Instructions

1. Melt the chocolate in a water bath or a stove pan on low heat while stirring, until fully melted and smooth.
2. In a medium-sized bowl, blend the silken tofu with a handheld mixer (a blender would work, too, but the handheld mixer makes it foamier).
3. Add the melted chocolate to the tofu and blend with the handheld mixer until fully combined and smooth.
4. Refrigerate (ideally for at least 24 hours before serving). If you prepare the mousse 1–3 days ahead of time, the flavors will unfold throughout the chilling process and you will get an even more flavorsome mousse. As this dessert is quite rich, try to keep your serving portions moderate in size.

Note: As a rule of thumb, you need 2 units of silken tofu to 1 unit of dark chocolate. You can play around with the cacao content of the dark chocolate; if you choose a higher cacao content, it will be less sweet. For me, a cacao content of 60% has proved to be the most convincing.

Sweet Cherry Ice Cream with Chocolate Sauce

Recipe by Marlene Watson-Tara

Ingredients

For the ice cream
- 2 cups frozen sweet cherries
- 2 cups banana, sliced
- 2 Tbsp plant-based milk
- 1/4 tsp vanilla extract

For the chocolate sauce
- 1/4 cup date or rice syrup
- 3 Tbsp cacao powder
- 1/2 tsp vanilla extract or powder

Instructions

For the ice cream
1. Peel and slice the bananas and freeze them in a freezer bag overnight.
2. Remove the bananas from the bag and allow them to sit on the countertop for a few minutes before processing. Place all the ingredients in a food processor or high-speed blender. Process until thick and creamy.
3. Serve immediately with the chocolate sauce and/or some fresh fruit.

Note: If using a blender, start slowly and increase the speed, using the tamper to push down the frozen fruit. Increase the speed to high, and continue to use the tamper by pushing the ingredients down to the blade. Blend until you reach a thick and creamy texture. You can add other berries and frozen fruits for beautiful colors and different tastes.

For the chocolate sauce
1. In a small bowl, mix all the ingredients together. Pour into a squeezy bottle and use it as a decorative treat for ice cream or other desserts. Keep refrigerated.

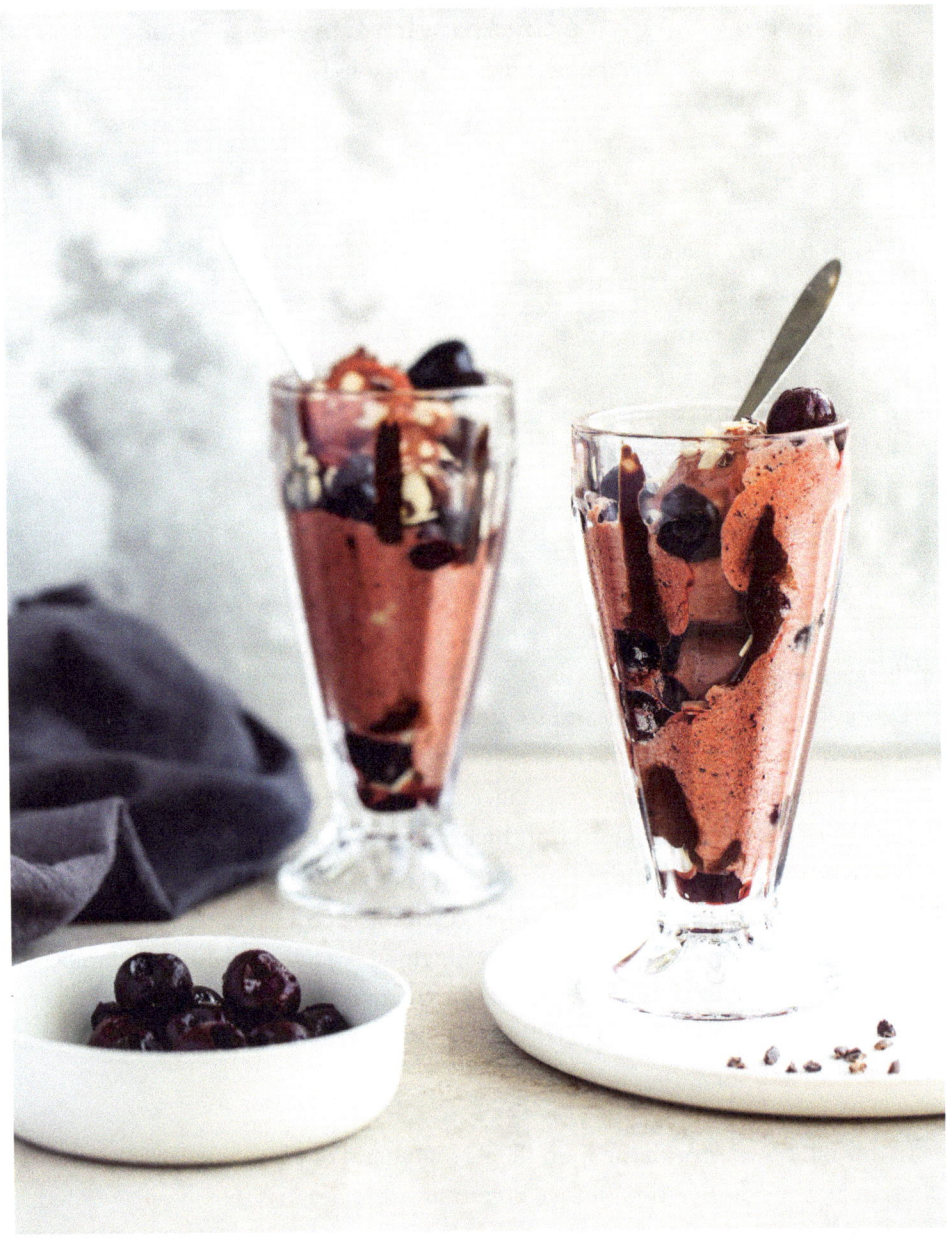

Source: Go Vegan (Lotus Publishing, 2019).

Baked Banana
Recipe by Jim McGehee

Ingredients
- 1 banana per person

Instructions
1. Peel bananas and slice them half lengthwise.
2. Place them on a baking sheet (without silicone mat or parchment paper) and broil. Check after 10 minutes and watch carefully.

Coconut Kisses
Recipe by Camila Perussello

Ingredients
- 320 g (11 oz-can) sweetened plant-based condensed milk (preferably made of coconut milk)
- 1 Tbsp unsalted vegan butter
- 150 g (1 cup) shredded coconut (sweetened or unsweetened, as preferred)
- Extra shredded coconut for rolling the balls
- Cloves for decorating

Instructions
1. In a saucepan, combine the condensed milk, butter, and shredded coconut. Cook the mixture over medium heat, stirring constantly to prevent it from sticking to the bottom of the pan. Keep stirring until the mixture thickens and starts to pull away from the sides of the pan. This usually takes about 10–15 minutes.
2. Remove the pan from the heat and let the mixture cool down until you can handle it comfortably with your hands. If necessary, use the fridge to speed up the cooling process.
3. Roll small portions of the mixture into small balls (about 1 inch in diameter) using the palms of your hands. If the mixture is too sticky, grease your hands lightly with vegan butter or oil.

4. Roll each ball in additional shredded coconut to coat them evenly. The coconut flakes will stick to the outside of the balls, giving them a nice texture.
5. Stick one clove into the top of each ball for a beautiful finish (and extra flavor). Place the coconut balls on a nice plate or tray. They can be served immediately or refrigerated for a firmer texture. If you prepare the sweets one day ahead of serving, they will develop even richer flavors.

Note: You can place each coconut kiss inside a mini cupcake liner or mini baking cup for a festive look. These paper trays come in various colors, patterns, and sizes, adding a decorative touch to party displays.

Oatmeal Walnut Cookies
Recipe by Marlene Watson-Tara

Ingredients
- 1 1/2 cups oatmeal
- 90 g (3/4 cup) whole-wheat pastry flour
- 90 g (3/4 cup) unbleached white flour or almond flour
- 1 tsp baking powder
- 1/4 tsp sea salt
- 3/4 cup currants
- 1 cup walnuts, toasted and coarsely chopped
- 2 Tbsp apple butter
- 1/2 cup barley malt or brown rice syrup
- Zest of 1 orange
- 1/2 cup orange juice
- 1 Tbsp finely grated fresh ginger
- 1 tsp vanilla

Instructions

1. Preheat the oven to 170°C (338°F), gas 4. Line two baking trays with parchment paper.
2. In a large bowl, mix the dry ingredients. In a smaller bowl, whisk together the wet ingredients and then stir into the dry ingredients.
3. Transfer heaping tablespoons of dough to the baking sheet, leaving at least 1 inch (2 cm) of space between the cookies. Flatten the cookies with the back of a fork to make rounds. Dip the fork in water to keep the mixture from sticking.
4. Bake the cookies until the edges and undersides are golden, for 20–25 minutes. Remove from the oven and allow to cool on a rack.

Makes 16–18 cookies.

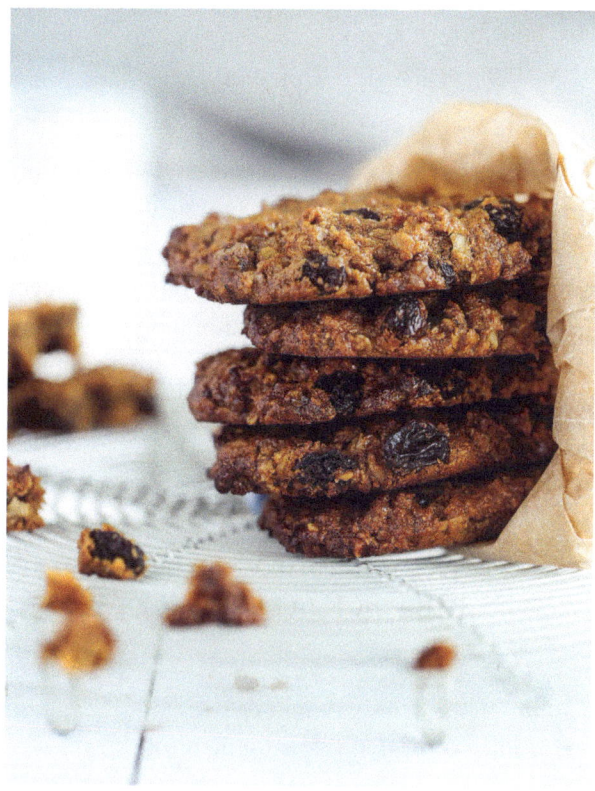

Source: Go Vegan (Lotus Publishing, 2019).

Blueberry & Banana Muffins
Recipe by Fernando Grando

Ingredients
- 200 g (1 1/2 cups) blueberries (fresh)
- 2 ripe bananas (reserve a portion for the topping)
- 200 g (7 oz) all-purpose flour
- 3 Tbsp ground flaxseed
- 60 mL (1/4 cup) water
- 1/2 Tbsp baking powder
- 100 mL (approximately 1/2 cup) oat milk
- 80 mL (1/3 cup) sunflower oil
- 100 g (3 1/2 oz) light brown sugar
- 50 g (1 3/4 oz) walnuts or pecan nuts, chopped

Instructions
1. Whisk the ground flaxseed with water and set aside for 5 minutes.
2. In the meantime, smash one and a half bananas with a fork and cut the blueberries in half. Slice the remaining banana thinly and set aside.
3. In a big bowl, mix the flaxseed mixture, mashed bananas, blueberries, sunflower oil, oat milk, sugar, chopped nuts, flour, and baking powder.
4. Distribute the dough into silicone muffin molds with a spoon. Top each muffin with a thin banana slice and, optionally, a sprinkle of sugar.
5. Bake at 180°C for 20–25 minutes. These are supposed to be fluffy and moist muffins, so watch out not to overbake them.

Lemon Tofu Mousse
Recipe by Karoline Mueller

Ingredients
- 450 g (16-oz) tofu
- Zest of lemon, or juice of 1 lemon if using firm tofu
- 1/2–1 tsp vanilla extract
- Sweetener to taste: ~ 1 or less Tbsp sugar or 2 Tbsp date paste

Instructions

Tofu comes in a range of consistencies. Blend as follows:
1. If you are using a regular blender, buy silken tofu and blend with zest of half a lemon, 1/2 tsp vanilla extract, and sweetener.
2. If using a high-powered blender, extra-firm tofu can be worked into a smooth mousse. Squeeze out the water first. In the blender, combine tofu with lemon zest and juice, 1 tsp vanilla extract, and sweetener to taste.

Mini Orange Chocolate Cups
Recipe by Marlene Watson-Tara

Ingredients
- 120 g (4 oz) 100% cocoa chocolate
- 300 g (10 1/2 oz) pack organic silken tofu
- 1/4 cup maple syrup
- 1/4 cup rice milk
- 1 tsp lemon juice
- 1 heaped Tbsp tahini
- 1/4 tsp pure orange extract
- 1/4 tsp vanilla extract
- Fresh orange slices, to serve
- Desiccated coconut for garnish

Instructions
1. Put a small amount of boiling filtered water in a saucepan. Place a metal bowl on top of the pan. Break the chocolate into pieces in the metal bowl and stir until melted. Remove from the heat.
2. In a blender, purée all ingredients to a cream. Divide into small cups and chill in the refrigerator until set. Serve with a few fresh orange slices and garnish with desiccated coconut.

Makes 6 servings.

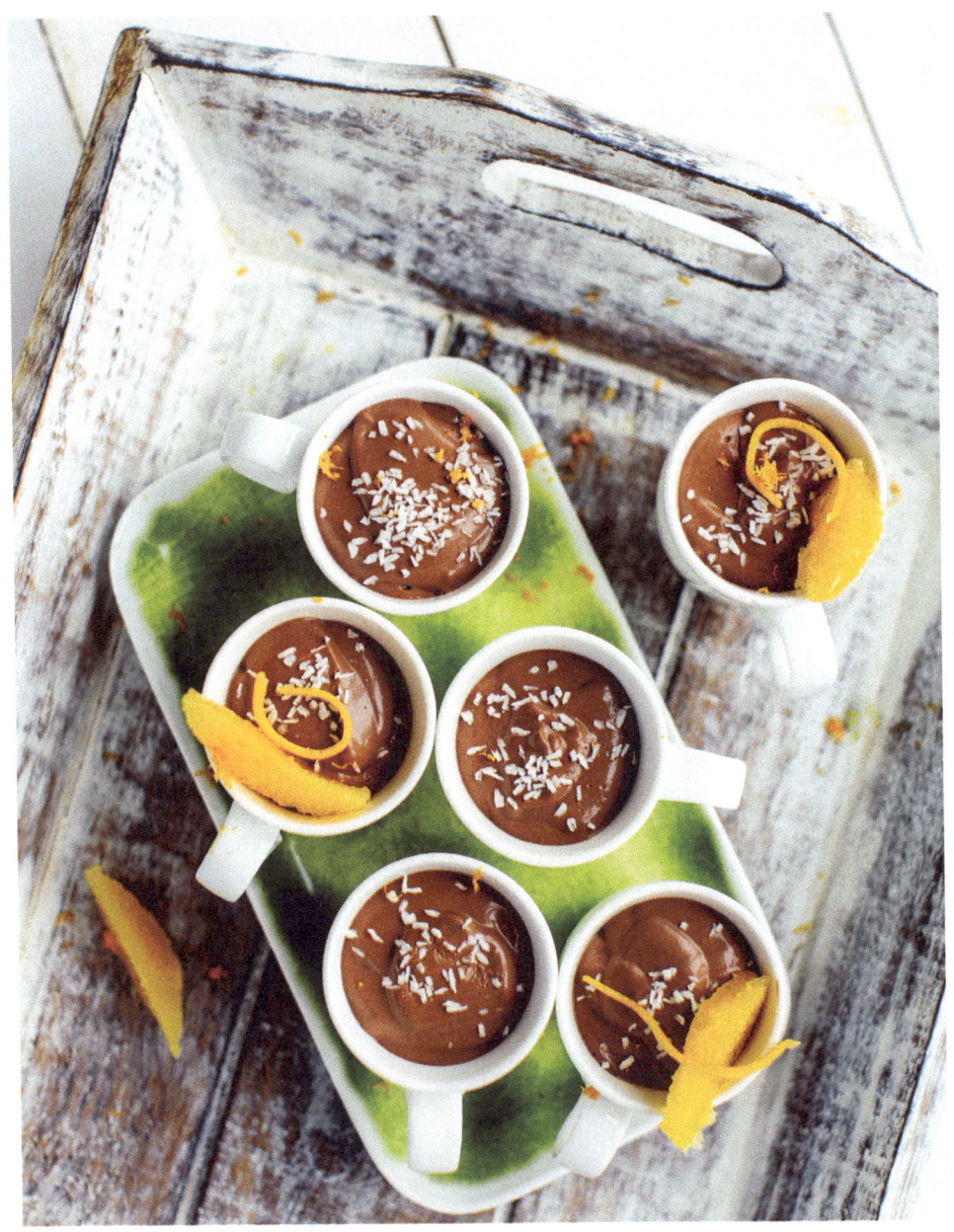

Source: Go Vegan (Lotus Publishing, 2019).

Chapter 7

Resources

The aim of this book is to give readers an overview of why and how to be vegan. As discussed throughout these pages, veganism is a social justice movement that emphasizes the complete cessation of animal use for any purpose, including food, clothing, research, and entertainment. This chapter suggests books, documentaries, websites, podcasts, and apps that may help you gain a deeper knowledge of veganism and make your transition to plant-based living smooth and uncomplicated. This section also contains resources to help you connect with like-minded people and lead a happier and more fulfilling life.

When exploring these resources, keep in mind that different activists and organizations may have varying approaches and focuses within the broader scope of animal rights. It is advisable to explore multiple sources to gain a comprehensive understanding of the animal liberation movement and how to accelerate our common goal.

Please note that we have *not* included websites for vegan sanctuaries to avoid giving the impression that we favor some over others. Numerous vegan sanctuaries around the world play a crucial role in rescuing, rehabilitating, and providing lifelong care to animals saved from exploitation. With their dedication to animal rescue and advocacy, these sanctuaries contribute significantly to changing perceptions about nonhuman animals and advancing a society where the rights of other individuals are taken seriously. Whatever their size and capacity, multiple animal sanctuaries are doing valuable work worldwide.

While this chapter is not an exhaustive list of resources on veganism, it will give you a glimpse of the wealth of valuable information available. Being vegan is easy; all that it takes is for you to care.

7.1 Books

- *Animal Factories* by Jim Mason and Peter Singer
- *Animal Liberation* by Peter Singer
- *Beyond Beliefs: A Guide to Improving Relationships and Communication for Vegans, Vegetarians, and Meat Eaters* by Melanie Joy, PhD
- *Eat for the Planet: Saving the World One Bite at a Time* by Nil Zacharias and Gene Stone
- *Eating Animals* by Jonathan Safran Foer
- *Eat Like You Care: An Examination of the Morality of Eating Animals* by Gary L. Francione and Anna Charlton
- *The Face on Your Plate: The Truth About Food* by Jeffrey Moussaieff Masson
- *Farm Sanctuary: Changing Hearts and Minds About Animals and Food* by Gene Baur
- *Food for Thought: Planetary Healing Begins on Our Plate* by Camila Perussello, PhD
- *Food Is Climate* by Glen Merzer
- *The Food Revolution: How Your Diet Can Help Save Your Life and Our World* by John Robbins
- *Forks Over Knives: The Plant-Based Way to Health*, by Gene Stone, T. Colin Campbell, and Caldwell B. Esselstyn
- *The Future of Nutrition* by T. Colin Campbell, PhD
- *How Not to Die* and *How Not to Diet* by Dr. Michael Greger
- *How to Create a Vegan World* by Tobias Leenaert
- *The Humane Hoax: Essays Exposing the Myth of Happy Meat, Humane Dairy, and Ethical Eggs*, edited by Hope Bohanec
- *The Joyful Vegan* by Colleen Patrick Goudreau
- *Letters to a New Vegan: Words to Inform, Inspire, and Support a Vegan Lifestyle* by Lantern
- *Mind If I Order the Cheeseburger?* by Sherry F. Colb
- *This Is Vegan Propaganda: (And Other Lies the Meat Industry Tells You)* by Ed Winters
- *The Ultimate Betrayal: Is There Happy Meat?* by Hope Bohanec with Cogen Bohanec
- *An Unnatural Order* by Jim Mason
- *A Vegan Ethic* by Mark Hawthorne
- *Vegan Voices: Essays by Inspiring Changemakers*, edited by Dr. Joanne Kong
- *Vystopia: The Anguish of Being Vegan in a Non-vegan World* by Clare Mann
- *We Animals* by Jo-Anne McArthur
- *Why We Love Dogs, Eat Pigs, and Wear Cows: An Introduction to Carnism* by Melanie Joy, PhD
- *The World Peace Diet* by Will Tuttle, PhD

7.2 Documentaries

- *Meet Your Meat* (2002, 12 minutes)
- *Peaceable Kingdom* (2004)
- *Earthlings* (2005)
- *Food, Inc.* (2008)
- *Forks Over Knives* (2011)
- *Vegucated* (2011)
- *Live and Let Live* (2013)
- *Speciesism* (2013)
- *Cowspiracy* (2014)
- *Plant Pure Nation* (2015)
- *Unity* (2015)
- *What Cody Saw* (2015, 11 minutes)
- *Eating You Alive* (2016)
- *Food Choices* (2016)
- *Eating Animals* (2017)
- *The End of Meat* (2017)
- *What the Health* (2017)
- *Dominion* (2018)
- *The Game Changers* (2018)
- *Prayer for Compassion* (2018)
- *Gunda* (2020)
- *Cow* (2021)
- *Eating Our Way to Extinction* (2021)
- *Seaspiracy* (2021)
- *They're Trying to Kill Us* (2021)
- *The Land of Ahimsa* (2022)
- *Live to 100: Secrets of the Blue Zones* (2023)
- *You Are What You Eat: A Twin Experiment* (2024)
- *Christspiracy (2024)*
- *Pignorant (2024)*

7.3 Websites

- *7dayvegan.com*
    A guide to going vegan, with meal plans, nutrition info, inspiring stories, and more.
- *abolitionistapproach.com*
    The Abolitionist Approach, founded by Prof. Gary L. Francione, promotes veganism as a moral baseline and provides resources to support individuals in adopting and promoting abolitionist veganism.
- *agriculturefairnessalliance.org*
    USA-based non-profit Agriculture Fairness Alliance (AFA) lobbies for veganism and fairness in Washington, DC.
- *aldf.org*
    The Animal Legal Defense Fund (ALDF) focuses on using the legal system to protect the fundamental rights of animals.
- *challenge22.com*
    Free online guidance by mentors and registered dietitians to help people become vegan.
- *chooseveg.com*
    Free plant-based recipes and nutrition tips, in addition to help for businesses looking to increase their plant-based options.
- *climatehealers.org*
    Climate Healers is a USA-based non-profit founded by systems engineer Dr. Sailesh Rao. They look to advance a vegan world by educating people on animal rights and the close relationship between animal exploitation and the climate crisis.
- *elwooddogmeat.com*
    Elwood's Organic Dog Meat is an animal advocacy initiative that draws attention to the moral inconsistencies among non-vegans.
- *findveglove.com*
    Matchmaking services to help vegetarian and vegan singles across North America find a partner.
- *thefirstmess.com*
    Delicious vegan recipes with a focus on wholesome and seasonal meals.
- *goveganworld.com*
    Go Vegan World is an Ireland-based animal rights and advocacy organization. Their website covers a wide range of topics on the intersectional harms caused by animal use, including a section on the rights of vegans.
- *hercampus.com/school/clemson/how-eat-vegan-college-dining-hall*
    Her Campus is an online magazine targeted at the female college student demographic, which has an interesting article on eating vegan in universities.

- *howdoigovegan.com*
    Created by the same founder as The Abolitionist Approach, this website serves as a practical guide to transitioning to a vegan lifestyle based on abolitionist principles.
- *makeitdairyfree.com*
    Plant-based recipes, product reviews, and food shopping guide.
- *nonhumanrights.org*
    The Nonhuman Rights Project is an organization dedicated to securing legally recognized fundamental rights for nonhuman animals.
- *nutritionfacts.org*
    The latest science about diet and health by plant-based physician Dr. Michael Greger.
- *pcrm.org/veganstarterkit*
    The Physicians Committee for Responsible Medicine offers a free booklet to help people transition to plant-based eating.
- *plantbasedonabudget.com*
    Tasty, affordable, and easy-to-make plant-based recipes.
- *rainbowplantlife.com*
    Amazing vegan recipes and healthy lifestyle content.
- *theminimalistvegan.com*
    Website that inspires people to live vegan and with less stuff.
- *vegan.com/info/how*
    This guide explains how to go vegan with minimal effort in a lasting and healthy way.
- *vegan.com/blog/sanctuaries*
    The Farm Animal Sanctuary Directory lists vegan sanctuaries in the United States and worldwide that provide a safe home for formerly farmed animals.
- *veganhealth.org*
    Nutrition tips for vegans.
- *veganlinked.com*
    Vegan Linked is a platform for vegan professionals to connect and promote their work.
- *veganproducts.org/vegan-ingredients*
    Vegan staples listed by class of ingredients.
- *vegansociety.com*
    The Vegan Society is the first vegan charity in the world. Their website covers everything from animal rights to lifestyle to statistics on veganism.
- *veggiedate.org*
    Considered one of the best vegetarian and vegan dating websites in the world.
- *viva.org.uk*
    Viva! is the United Kingdom's leading vegan charity, specializing in high-profile animal campaigns and undercover investigations exposing the reality of animal farming.

7.4 Podcasts

- Always for Animal Rights (radio show with Carolyn Harris)
- Chef AJ Live!
- The Exam Room Podcast (Chuck Carroll)
- Food for Thought with Colleen Patrick Goudreau
- The Glen Merzer Show: Real Men Eat Plants Podcast
- Hope for the Animals (Hope Bohanec)
- Main Street Vegan with Victoria Moran
- The Minimalist Vegan Podcast (Michael & Maša Ofei)
- No Meat Athlete (radio show with Matt Frazier)
- NutritionFacts Podcast with Michael Greger, M.D.
- Our Hen House (Jasmin Singer and Mariann Sullivan)
- The Plant-Based News Podcast (Robbie Lockie, Joe Best, Polly Foreman, and Klaus Mitchell)
- Plantstrong Podcast (Rip Esselstyn)
- Switch4Good (Dotsie Bausch and Alexandra Paul)
- The Rich Roll Podcast
- Unchained TV Video Podcast (Jane Velez-Mitchell)
- Vegan Mainstream (Stephanie Redcross West)
- Vegan Nation (radio show with Marlene Narrow)

7.5 Apps

- **21-Day Vegan Kickstart**: recipes and nutrition information.
- **Barnivore**: indicates whether alcoholic beverages are vegan.
- **Bunny Free (PETA)**: identifies if products are tested on animals.
- **Dr. Greger's Daily Dozen**: helps you keep track of daily servings of healthy foods.
- **Food Monster**: over 8,000 vegan recipes.
- **Forks Over Knives**: plant-based recipes and meal plans.
- **Grazer**: vegan dating app.
- **Happy Cow**: vegan-friendly restaurants and stores around the world.
- **Oh She Glows**: plant-based recipes, including dishes for special occasions.
- **So Vegan**: recipes with the option to export ingredients to a shopping list.
- **Vanilla Bean**: similar to Happy Cow.
- **Vegan Additives**: helps you determine if supermarket products are vegan.
- **Vegan Scan**: similar to Vegan Additives.
- **Vegan Sports Nutrition Guide**: explains how and what to eat for different activity levels, fitness goals, and sports.
- **Veggly**: dating app for vegetarians and vegans.
- **VeGuide app**: guide by the Vegan Society with everything you need to start your vegan journey.
- **VNutrition**: food intake tracker, food diary, and plant-based nutrition tips for pregnant and breastfeeding women.

Final Thoughts

Dr. Camila Perussello

As we wrap up this journey through the pages of our book, we are filled with a profound sense of purpose and hope. Our drive to create this guide stemmed from a firm conviction in the transformative power of veganism—not just as a diet but as the tipping point for a society that takes justice and ethics seriously.

This work demanded considerable time and effort, not only from us, the authors, but from all those engaged in bringing this content to you, encompassing endorsers, designers, chefs, editors, publishers, and other contributors. On our part, countless hours were devoted to meticulous research, writing, and in-depth discussions, ensuring the information presented is accurate, comprehensive, and accessible. We aimed to turn our knowledge and experience into practical, easy-to-follow guidance. From conceptualization to completion, every chapter reflects our dedication to our fellow animals and our sincere desire to provide readers with a meaningful resource for a compassionate and sustainable lifestyle.

This book is a tribute to the countless beings who endure unimaginable suffering and meet untimely ends each year, victims of a system that overlooks their sentience. We earnestly hope this work inspires readers to take concrete action, embracing the empathy, peace, and unity that only veganism brings. May this book illuminate our path toward a more mindful and ethical existence where our choices reflect respect for other living beings.

References

Aghasi, M.; Golzarand, M.; Shab-Bidar, S.; et al. (2019). Dairy intake and acne development: A meta-analysis of observational studies. Clinical Nutrition, 38(3):1067–75.

Baker, K. (2018). Counting calories? Count your carbon, too. Columbia University Mailman School of Public Health, www.publichealth.columbia.edu/news/counting-calories-count-your-carbon-too.

Bar-On, Y. M.; Milo, R.; Phillips, R. (2018). The biomass distribution on Earth. *Proceedings of the National Academy of Sciences,* 115(25):6506–11.

Barnard, N. (2020). Your body in balance: The new science of food, hormones, and health. New York, USA: Hachette Book Group.

Berners-Lee, M.; Kennelly, C.; Watson, R.; Hewitt, C. N. (2018). Current global food production is sufficient to meet human nutritional needs in 2050 provided there is radical societal adaptation. Elementa: Science of the Anthropocene, 6:52.

Braesco, V.; Souchon, I.; Sauvant, P.; et al. (2022). Ultra-processed foods: How functional is the NOVA system? European Journal of Clinical Nutrition, 76:1245–53.

Bunner, A.; Agarwal, U.; Gonzales, J.; Valente, F.; Barnard, N. (2014). Nutrition intervention for migraine: A randomized crossover trial. The Journal of Headache and Pain, 15:69.

Campbell, T. C.; Campbell II, T. M. (2005). The China study. New York, USA: BenBella.

Cao, Y.; Liu, H.; Qin, N.; et al. (2020). Impact of food additives on the composition and function of gut microbiota: A review. Trends in Food Science & Technology, 99:295–310.

Carrington, D. (2023). "Gigantic" power of meat industry blocking green alternatives, study finds. The Guardian, https://www.theguardian.com/environment/2023/aug/18/gigantic-power-of-meat-industry-blocking-green-alternatives-study-finds.

CBS News (2022). As America's milk consumption declines, some farmers find alternatives, www.cbsnews.com/news/milk-consumption-dairy-farmers/.

Chavez, G. N.; Jaworsky, K.; Basu, A. (2023). The effects of plant-derived phytochemical compounds and phytochemical-rich diets on females with polycystic ovarian syndrome: A scoping review of clinical trials. International Journal of Environmental Research and Public Health, 20(15):6534.

Chen, X.; Zhang, Z.; Yang, H.; et al. (2020). Consumption of ultra-processed foods and health outcomes: A systematic review of epidemiological studies. Nutrition Journal, 19:86.

Clark, M.; Tilman, D. (2017). Comparative analysis of environmental impacts of agricultural production systems, agricultural input efficiency, and food choice. Environmental Research Letters, 12:064016.

Cordova, R.; Viallon, V.; Fontvieille, E.; et al. (2023). Consumption of ultra-processed foods and risk of multimorbidity of cancer and cardiometabolic diseases: a multinational cohort study. The Lancet – Regional Health Europe, 35:100771.

DeClercq, V.; Nearing, J. T.; Sweeney, E. (2022). Plant-based diets and cancer risk: What is the evidence?. Current Nutrition Reports, 11:354–69.

Derbyshire, E. (2019). Are all "ultra-processed" foods nutritional demons? A commentary and nutritional profiling analysis. Trends in Food Science & Technology, 94:98–104.

Dimitras, E. (2021). Everything you need to know about animal testing. Ethos & Empathy, www.ethosandempathy.org/en/2021/06/21/everything-you-need-to-know-about-animal-testing/.

Ding, H.; Reiss, A. B.; Pinkhasov, A.; et al. (2022). Plants, plants, and more plants: Plant-derived nutrients and their protective roles in cognitive function, Alzheimer's disease, and other dementias. Medicina, 58:1025.

Dunneram, Y.; Greenwood, D. C.; Cade, J. E. (2019). Diet and risk of breast, endometrial and ovarian cancer: UK Women's Cohort Study. British Journal of Nutrition, 122(5):564–74.

Eisen, M. B.; Brown, P. O. (2022). Rapid global phaseout of animal agriculture has the potential to stabilize greenhouse gas levels for 30 years and offset 68 percent of CO_2 emissions this century. PLOS Climate, 1(2):e0000010.

FAO – Food and Agriculture Organization of the United Nations. (2006). Livestock's long shadow – Environmental issues and options, www.fao.org/3/a0701e/a0701e00.htm.

FAO – Food and Agriculture Organization of the United Nations. (2013). World Livestock 2013: Changing disease landscapes, www.fao.org/3/i3440e/i3440e.pdf.

FAO – Food and Agriculture Organization of the United Nations. (2023). The state of food and agriculture 2023 – Revealing the true cost of food to transform agrifood systems, https://www.fao.org/documents/card/en/c/cc7724en.

Finelli, M. (2021). Swimming against ignorance and cruelty, in Vegan voices: Essays by inspiring changemakers, Kong, J., ed. New York, USA: Lantern Publishing & Media.

Foer, J. S. (2009). Eating animals. New York, USA: Little, Brown and Company.

Francione, G. (2022). Animal welfare and society—part 1, The viewpoints of a philosopher. Animal Frontiers, www.academic.oup.com/af/article/12/1/43/6550174.

Francione, G. (undated). Animal rights: The abolitionist approach, www.abolitionistapproach.com/quotes/.

Fusano, M. (2023). Veganism in acne, atopic dermatitis, and psoriasis: Benefits of a plant-based diet. Clinics in Dermatology, 41(1):122–26.

Gardner, C. D.; Hartle, J. C.; Garrett, R. D.; et al. (2019). Maximizing the intersection of human health and the health of the environment with regard to the amount and type of protein produced and consumed in the United States. Nutrition Reviews, 77(4):197–215.

Goodland, R.; Anhang, J. (2009). Livestock and climate change: What if the key actors in climate change are . . . cows, pigs, and chickens? World Watch Magazine, pp.10–19 (Washington, D.C: Worldwatch Institute).

Greenpeace (undated). Overfishing & destructive fishing, www.greenpeace.org/usa/oceans/issues/overfishing-destructive-fishing/.

Greger, M. (2015). How not to die: Discover the foods scientifically proven to prevent and reverse disease. New York, USA: Flatiron Books.

Guéraud, F.; Héliès-Toussaint, C.; Dupuy, J.; et al. (2024). Meat and digestive cancers, in Encyclopedia of meat sciences, 3d ed., Dikeman, M., ed., pp.684–94. Amsterdam, Netherlands: Elsevier.

Harwatt, H.; Wetterberg, K.; Girithiran, A.; Benton, T. G. (2022). Aligning food systems with climate and diversity targets: Assessing the suitability of policy action over the next decade. London: Royal Institute of International Affairs, https://doi.org/10.55317/9781784135416.

Hayek, M. N.; Harwatt, H.; Ripple, W. J.; Mueller, N. D. (2020). The carbon opportunity cost of animal-sourced food production on land. Nature Sustainability, 4:21–4.

Heaney, R. P.; Weaver, S. M.; Hinders, B.; et al. (1993). Absorbability of calcium from Brassica vegetables: Broccoli, bok choy, and kale. Journal of Food Science, 58(6):1378–80.

Herpich, C.; Müller-Werdan, U.; Norman, K. (2022). Role of plant-based diets in promoting health and longevity. Maturitas, 165:47–51.

Huang, Y.; Cao, D.; Chen, Z.; et al. (2021). Red and processed meat consumption and cancer outcomes: Umbrella review. Food Chemistry, 356:129697.

IPCC – Intergovernmental Panel on Climate Change (2019). An IPCC special report on climate change, desertification, land degradation, sustainable land management, food security, and greenhouse gas fluxes in terrestrial ecosystems, https://www.ipcc.ch/site/assets/uploads/2019/08/Fullreport-1.pdf.

Kahleova, H.; Levin, S.; Barnard, N. (2017). Cardio-metabolic benefits of plant-based diets. Nutrients, 9(8):848.

Kassam, S.; Kassam, Z. (2022). Eating plant-based: Scientific answers to your nutrition questions. London, UK: Hammersmith Health Books.

Kim, H.; Rebholz, C.; Hegde, S.; et al. (2021). Plant-based diets, pescatarian diets and COVID-19 severity: A population-based case–control study in six countries. BMJ Nutrition, Prevention & Health, 4(1):257–66.

Knorr, D.; Augustin, M. A. (2021). Food processing needs, advantages and misconceptions. Trends in Food Science & Technology, 108:103–10.

Lakhani, N. (2023). US dairy policies drive small farms to "get big or get out" as monopolies get rich. The Guardian, https://www.theguardian.com/environment/2023/jan/31/us-dairy-policies-hurt-small-farms-monopolies-get-rich.

Łakoma, K.; Kukharuk, O.; Śliż, D. (2023). The influence of metabolic factors and diet on fertility. Nutrients, 15:1180.

Le, L.; Sabaté, J. (2014). Beyond meatless, the health effects of vegan diets: Findings from the Adventist cohorts. Nutrients, 6:2131–47.

Leatherby, L.; Merrill, D. (2018). Here's how America uses its land. Bloomberg, www.bloomberg.com/graphics/2018-us-land-use/.

Li, Y.; Liao, L. M.; Sinha, R.; et al. (2022). Fish intake and risk of melanoma in the NIH-AARP diet and health study. Cancer Causes Control, 33:921–8.

Lockwood, A. (2021). How COP26 almost brought me to tears, www.sunderland.ac.uk/more/news/story/university-expert-how-cop26-almost-brought-me-to-tears-1695.

Lucas, E.; Guo, M.; Guillén-Gosálbez, G. (2023). Low-carbon diets can reduce global ecological and health costs. Nature Foods, 4:394–406.

Mann, C. (2018). Vystopia: The anguish of being vegan in a non-vegan world. Sydney, Australia: Communicate31.

Mason, J. (2021). An unnatural order: The roots of our destruction of nature. New York, USA: Lantern Publishing & Media.

Matsushita, M.; Fujita, K.; Hatano, K.; et al. (2023). Emerging relationship between the gut microbiome and prostate cancer. World Journal of Men's Health, 41(4):759–68.

McCarthy, J.; Sánchez, E. (2018). The earth needs 5 million years to recover from humans. Global Citizen, www.globalcitizen.org/en/content/earth-5-million-years-to-recover/#:~:text=Using%20advanced%20modeling%20programs%20and,seen%20prior%20to%20human%20life.

Mekonnen, M. M.; Hoekstra, A. Y. (2010). The green, blue and grey water footprint of farm animals and animal products. UNESCO – IHE Institute for Water Education. Research Report Series No. 48.

Melina, V.; Craig, W.; Levin, S. (2016). Position of the Academy of Nutrition and Dietetics: Vegetarian diets. Journal of the Academy of Nutrition and Dietetics, 116(12):1970–80.

Melnik, B. C.; John, S. M.; Carrera-Bastos, P.; et al. (2023). The role of cow's milk consumption in breast cancer initiation and progression. Current Nutrition Reports, 12:122–40.

Melse-Boonstra, A. (2020). Bioavailability of micronutrients from nutrient-dense whole foods: Zooming in on dairy, vegetables, and fruits. Frontiers in Nutrition, 7.

Menzel, J.; Jabakhanji, A.; Biemann, R.; et al. (2020). Systematic review and meta-analysis of the associations of vegan and vegetarian diets with inflammatory biomarkers. Nature Scientific Reports, 10:21736.

Micha, R.; Khatibzadeh, S.; Shi, P. (2014). Global, regional, and national consumption levels of dietary fats and oils in 1990 and 2010: A systematic analysis including 266 country-specific nutrition surveys BMJ, 348:g2272.

Mills, M. (2020). Dairy is not a health food. Switch4Good Podcast, www.youtube.com/watch?v=StevqYf_7T4.

Miranda, R de.; Weimer, P.; Rossi, R.C. (2021). Effects of hydrolyzed collagen supplementation on skin aging: A systematic review and meta-analysis. International Journal of Dermatology, 60(12):1449–61.

Mobasheri, A.; Mahmoudian, A.; Kalvaityte, U.; et al. (2021). A white paper on collagen hydrolyzates and ultrahydrolyzates: Potential supplements to support joint health in osteoarthritis? Current Rheumatology Reports, 23(78).

Monteiro, C.A. (2009). Nutrition and health. The issue is not food, nor nutrients, so much as processing. Public Health Nutrition, 12(5): 729–31.

Mridul, A. (2021). Exclusive: 56% of American vegans wouldn't date meat-eaters. The Vegan Review, www.theveganreview.com/exclusive-56-percent-of-american-vegans-wouldnt-date-meat-eaters-relationship/.

Muhammed, N., interview by Goodman, A. (2017). North Carolina hog farms spray manure around black communities; Residents fight back, www.democracynow.org/2017/5/3/nc_lawmakers_side_with_factory_farms.

Nath, P.; Singh, S. (2017). Chapter 26 – Defecation and stools in vegetarians: Implications in health and disease. In Vegetarian and plant-based diets in health and disease prevention, Mariotti, F., ed. Cambridge, USA: Academic Press.

Neufingerl, N.; Eilander, A. (2022). Nutrient intake and status in adults consuming plant-based diets compared to meat-eaters: A systematic review. Nutrients, 14(29).

NHS – National Health System of the United Kingdom (2023). Food colours and hyperactivity. https://www.nhs.uk/conditions/food-colours-and-hyperactivity/.

Open Sanctuary Staff. (2018). What should a sanctuary do with residents' eggs? Explore Open Sanctuary, www.opensanctuary.org/what-to-do-about-egg-laying/.

Pachirat, T. (2011). Every twelve seconds: Industrialized slaughter and the politics of sight. New Haven, USA: Yale University Press.

Perussello, C. (2022). Food for thought: Planetary healing begins on our plate. New York, USA: Lantern Publishing & Media.

Petrus, R. R.; Sobral, P. J. A.; Tadini, C. C.; et al. (2021). The NOVA classification system: A critical perspective in food science. Trends in Food Science & Technology, 116:603–8.

PAN – Physicians Association for Nutrition. (2023). PAN International's position paper on plant-based meat products. https://pan-int.org/plant-based-meat-position-paper/.

PCRM – Physicians Committee for Responsible Medicine. (undated). Health concerns with eggs: Eating eggs can be hazardous to your health, www.pcrm.org/good-nutrition/nutrition-information/health-concerns-with-eggs.

Pimentel, D. (1979). Food, energy, and society. New York, USA: John Wiley & Sons.

Poore, J.; Nemecek, T. (2018). Reducing food's environmental impacts through producers and consumers. Science, 360:987–92.

Ranganathan, J.; Vennard, D.; Waite, R.; et al. (2016). Shifting diets for a sustainable food future. Creating a sustainable food future, 11 (Washington, D.C.: World Resources Institute).

Rao, M.; Afshin, A.; Singh, G.; et al. (2013). Do healthier foods and diet patterns cost more than less healthy options? A systematic review and meta-analysis. BMJ Open, 3:e004277.

Rao, S. (2021). Animal agriculture is the leading cause of climate change – a position paper. Journal of the Ecological Society, 32–33:155–67.

Ravella, S. (2022). A silent fire: The story of inflammation, diet & disease. New York, USA: W.W. Norton.

Reisinger, A.; Clark, H. (2018). How much do direct livestock emissions actually contribute to global warming? Global Change Biology, 24(4):1749–61.

Ritchie, H. (2020). You want to reduce the carbon footprint of your food? Focus on what you eat, not whether your food is local. Our World in Data, https://ourworldindata.org/food-choice-vs-eating-local.

Ritchie, H. (2021a). If the world adopted a plant-based diet we would reduce global agricultural land use from 4 to 1 billion hectares. Our World in Data: https://ourworldindata.org/land-use-diets.

Ritchie, H. (2021b). Cutting down forests: What are the drivers of deforestation? Our World in Data, www.ourworldindata.org/what-are-drivers-deforestation.

Ryan, R. (2022). The survival of the egg industry in Ireland at risk. Irish Examiner, https://www.irishexaminer.com/farming/arid-40951334.html.

Sakkas, H.; Bozidis, P.; Touzios, C.; et al. (2020). Nutritional status and the influence of the vegan diet on the gut microbiota and human health. Medicina (Kaunas), 56(2):88.

Scarborough, P.; Clark, M.; Cobiac, L.; Papier, K.; Knuppel, A.; Lynch, J.; Harrington, R.; Key, T.; Springmann, M. (2023). Vegans, vegetarians, fish-eaters and meat-eaters in the UK show discrepant environmental impacts. Nature Food, 4:565–74.

Skoracka, K.; Eder, P.; Łykowska-Szuber, L.; et al. (2020). Diet and nutritional factors in male (in)fertility—Underestimated factors. *Journal of Clinical Medicine*, 9(5):1400.

Silvan, L. (2021). Beyond joy, in Vegan voices: Essays by inspiring changemakers, Kong, J., ed. New York, USA: Lantern Publishing & Media.

Simon, D. (2013). Meatonomics: How the rigged economics of meat and dairy make you consume too much—and how to eat better, live longer, and spend smarter. Newburyport, USA: Conari Press.

Springmann, M.; Clark, M.; Mason-D'Croz, D.; et al. (2018a). Options for keeping the food system within environmental limits. Nature, 562:519–25.

Springmann, M.; Wiebe, K.; Mason-D'Croz, D.; et al. (2018b). Health and nutritional aspects of sustainable diet strategies and their association with environmental impacts: a global modelling analysis with country-level detail. Lancet Planet Health, 2:e451–61.

Springmann, M.; Clark, M. A.; Rayner, M.; et al. (2021). The global and regional costs of healthy and sustainable dietary patterns: A modelling study. The LANCET – Planetary Health, 5(11): E797–E807.

Springmann, M.; Van Dingenen, R.; Vandyck, T.; et al. (2023). The global and regional air quality impacts of dietary change. Nature Communications, 14:6227.

Steele, E. M.; Baraldi, L. G.; Louzada, M. L. D. C; et al. (2016). Ultra-processed foods and added sugars in the US diet: Evidence from a nationally representative cross-sectional study. BMJ Open, 6(3).

Terraseed (2022). Animal and environmental impacts of the supplement industry, cdn.shopify.com/s/files/1/0236/1117/9054/files/Environmental_and_Animal_Impacts_of_the_Supplement_Industry-Report_by_Terraseed.pdf?v=1657918048.

The Vegan Society. Definition of veganism, www.vegansociety.com/go-vegan/definition-veganism.

The World Counts (2023). Globally, we consume around 350 million tons of meat a year, www.theworldcounts.com/challenges/foods-and-beverages/world-consumption-of-meat.

Thomas, M. S.; Calle, M.; Fernandez, M. L. (2023). Healthy plant-based diets improve dyslipidemias, insulin resistance, and inflammation in metabolic syndrome. A narrative review. Advances in Nutrition, 14(1):44–54.

UNCCD – United Nations Convention to Combat Desertification (2022). Chronic land degradation: UN offers stark warnings and practical remedies in global land outlook 2, www.unccd.int/news-stories/press-releases/chronic-land-degradation-un-offers-stark-warnings-and-practical.

UNEP – United Nations Environmental Programme (2008). Fisheries subsidies: A critical issue for trade and sustainable development at the WTO: An introductory guide. UNEP, https://stg-wedocs.unep.org/bitstream/handle/20.500.11822/23020/Fisheries_Subsidies_Intro.pdf.

USDA – United States Department of Agriculture (2023). Chickens and eggs 2022 summary, downloads.usda.library.cornell.edu/usda-esmis/files/1v53jw96n/8g84p05lj/v692vk48g/ckegan23.pdf.

Vallone, S.; Lambin, E. F. (2023). Public policies and vested interests preserve the animal farming status quo at the expense of animal product analogs. One Earth, 6(9):1213–26.

VAN – Veganic Agriculture Network (2022). Veganic fertility: Growing plants from plants, https://www.goveganic.net/article205.html.

Vitale, K.; Hueglin, S. (2021). Update on vegetarian and vegan athletes: A review. Journal of Physical Fitness and Sports Medicine, 10(1):1–11.

Xu, M.; Rossi, K. L.; Campbell, G. L.; et al. (2016). Excess protein intake relative to fiber and cardiovascular events in elderly men with chronic kidney disease. Nutrition, Metabolism and Cardiovascular Diseases, 26(7):597–602.

Wang, T.; Masedunskas, A.; Willett, W. C.; et al. (2023). Vegetarian and vegan diets: Benefits and drawbacks, European Heart Journal, 44(36):3423–39.

WAP – World Animal Protection. (undated). Collateral damage: how factory farming drives up the use of toxic agricultural pesticides, www.worldanimalprotection.us/siteassets/reports-programmatic/collateral-damage-report.pdf.

Wasley, A.; Mendonça, E.; Youssef, Y.; Soutar, R. (2023). More than 800m Amazon trees felled in six years to meet beef demand. The Guardian, www.theguardian.com/environment/2023/jun/02/more-than-800m-amazon-trees-felled-in-six-years-to-meet-beef-demand.

Water Footprint Calculator (2023). Beef: The "king" of the big water footprints, www.water-calculator.org/news/articles/beef-king-big-water-footprints/#:~:text=In%20a%20country%20like%20the,keep%20up%20with%20the%20demand.

Weaver, C. M.; Heaney, R. P.; Connor, L.; et al. (2002). Bioavailability of calcium from tofu as compared with milk in premenopausal women. Journal of Food Science, 67(8):3144–47.

Weindl, I.; Popp, A.; Bodirsky, B. L.; et al. (2017). Livestock and human use of land: Productivity trends and dietary choices as drivers of future land and carbon dynamics. Global and Planetary Change, 159:1–10.

Whittleton, J. (2019). Chickens are one of the most abused animals on the planet. World Animal Protection, www.worldanimalprotection.org/latest/blogs/chickens-are-one-most-abused-animals-planet/.

WHO – World Health Organization & IARC – International Agency for Research on Cancer. (2015). IARC monographs evaluate consumption of red meat and processed meat. Press release n. 240 of 26 October 2015, www.iarc.who.int/wp-content/uploads/2018/07/pr240_E.pdf.

WHO – World Health Organization. (2019). Guideline: fortification of wheat flour with vitamins and minerals as a public health strategy. https://www.who.int/publications/i/item/9789240043398#:~:text=This%20guideline%20provides%20locally%20adaptable%2C%20clear%2C%20evidence-informed%20global,grounded%20in%20gender%2C%20equity%20and%20human%20rights%20approache.

WHO – World Health Organization. (2021). Cardiovascular diseases (CVDs). https://www.who.int/news-room/fact-sheets/detail/cardiovascular-diseases-(cvds).

WHO – World Health Organization. (2022). Cancer. https://www.who.int/news-room/fact-sheets/detail/cancer.

WHO – World Health Organization. (2023). Ninety-seventh meeting - Joint FAO/WHO Expert Committee on Food Additives (JECFA). https://www.who.int/publications/m/item/ninety-seventh-meeting-joint-fao-who-expert-committee-on-food-additives-(jecfa).

Woldeab, R. (2019). Industrialized meat production and land degradation: 3 reasons to shift to a plant-based diet, www.populationeducation.org/industrialized-meat-production-and-land-degradation-3-reasons-to-shift-to-a-plant-based-diet/#:~:text=In%20the%20U.S.%2C%20industrialized%20livestock%20production%20is%20directly,subject%20to%20extensive%20grazing%20without%20sufficient%20recovery%20periods.

Woo, L.; Lau, L.; Cheng, N.; et al. (2017). Efficacy of oral collagen in joint pain – Osteoarthritis and rheumatoid arthritis. Journal of Arthritis, 6(2):1000233.

World Economic Forum. (2021). Plant-based diets will be essential to the planet's future, report says, www.weforum.org/agenda/2021/02/plant-based-diet-biodiversity-report/.

Zang, E.; Jiang, L.; Cui, H.; et al. (2023). Only plant-based food additives: An overview on application, safety, and key challenges in the food industry. Food Reviews International, 39(8): 5132–63.

Zarantonello, D.; Brunori, G. (2023). The role of plant-based diets in preventing and mitigating chronic kidney disease: More light than shadows. Journal of Clinical Medicine, 12(19):6137.

Zhao, J.; Xu, L.; Sun, J.; et al. (2023). Global trends in incidence, death, burden and risk factors of early-onset cancer from 1990 to 2019. BMJ Oncology, 2:e000049.

Zhou, X.; Qiao, K.; Wu, H.; et al. (2023). The impact of food additives on the abundance and composition of gut microbiota. Molecules, 28:631.

About the Authors

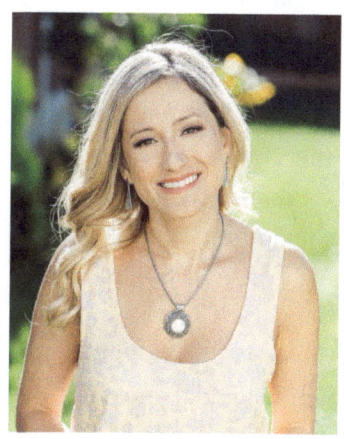

Dr. Camila Perussello, PhD, is an engineer, university lecturer and researcher specializing in bioprocessing engineering and sustainable food systems. She has published dozens of academic papers and book chapters on engineering, thermal sciences, and agrifood production topics, and serves as a peer-reviewer for over twenty renowned scientific journals. Her animal advocacy includes books, op-ed articles, multidisciplinary research, university teaching, and talks at academic and non-academic events. Dr. Perussello is also the author of *Food for Thought: Planetary Healing Begins on Our Plate* (Lantern Publishing & Media, 2022), the most comprehensive evidence-based book ever written on food production and animal rights. As an ethical vegan with expertise in food engineering, she promotes animal liberation through both educational and pragmatic solutions. Her academic research and industry consulting services aim to accelerate a sustainable and just food system by advancing the plant-based food sector and helping farmers and companies transition away from animal use. Find more information at www.camilaperussello.com.

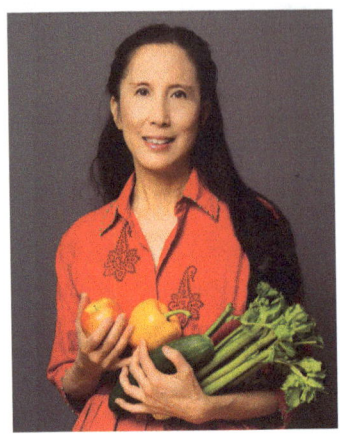

Dr. Joanne Kong, DMA, has been praised as one of the most compelling advocates for plant-based nutrition today, centered ethically in raising awareness that greater compassion for animals and our planet is vitally necessary for transformative growth and positive world change. Her TEDx talk, *The Power of Plant-Based Eating,* has over 1 million views on YouTube. She has appeared at numerous conferences and festivals, including the North American Veg Society Summerfest, San Francisco World Veg Fest, Veggie Pride Parade in New York City, National Animal Rights Day, VegFest Colorado, Twin Cities Veg Fest, Dr. Sailesh Rao's Vegan Convergence of the Peoples, Peace Advocacy Network, Compassion Arts Festival, the Physicians Committee for Responsible Medicine Plant-Based Climate Summit, and many others. Her vegan advocacy has been recognized around the world with international talks in Italy, Spain, Germany, Norway, Canada, and a three-week, ten-city tour of India. Dr. Kong is the editor of *Vegan Voices: Essays by Inspiring Changemakers* (Lantern Publishing & Media, 2021), which features fifty vegan advocates from around the world, is the author of *If You've Ever Loved an Animal, Go Vegan,* and was profiled in the book, *Legends of Change,* about vegan women impacting the world. She appears in the documentaries *Eating Our Way to Extinction* and *Taking Note.* Dr. Kong is a critically acclaimed, award-winning classical pianist on the music faculty at the University of Richmond and draws upon a diversity of skills as a musician, writer, speaker, and creative artist in her advocacy activities. Find further information on the websites www.vegansmakeadifference.com and www.joannekongmusic.com.

About the Publisher

Lantern Publishing & Media was founded in 2020 to follow and expand on the legacy of Lantern Books—a publishing company started in 1999 on the principles of living with a greater depth and commitment to the preservation of the natural world. Like its predecessor, Lantern Publishing & Media produces books on animal advocacy, veganism, religion, social justice, humane education, psychology, family therapy, and recovery. Lantern is dedicated to printing in the United States on recycled paper and saving resources in our day-to-day operations. Our titles are also available as ebooks and audiobooks.

To catch up on Lantern's publishing program, visit us at www.lanternpm.org.

facebook.com/lanternpm
instagram.com/lanternpm
tiktok.com/@lanternpmofficial